STRANGE AND DIFFICULT TIMES

T0038359

NANJALA NYABOLA

Strange and Difficult Times

Notes on a Global Pandemic

HURST & COMPANY, LONDON

First published in the United Kingdom in 2022 by
C. Hurst & Co. (Publishers) Ltd.,
New Wing, Somerset House, Strand, London, WC2R 1LA
Copyright © Nanjala Nyabola, 2022

All rights reserved.

The right of Nanjala Nyabola to be identified as the author of this publication is asserted by her in accordance with the Copyright, Designs and Patents Act, 1988.

Distributed in the United States, Canada and Latin America by
Oxford University Press, 198 Madison Avenue, New York, NY 10016,
United States of America.

A Cataloguing-in-Publication data record for this book
is available from the British Library.

ISBN: 9781787387805

A version of Chapter 3 was published by *Disegno* as "The Mask Generation" (2020). A version of Chapter 4 was published in *New Internationalist* as "View from Africa" (2020). A version of Chapter 5 was published in *The Nation* as "Africa Is Not Waiting to Be Saved From the Coronavirus" (2020). A version of Chapter 8 was published in Al Jazeera as "Police violence in the time of pandemic" (2020). A version of Chapter 10 was published in *Boston Review* as "How to Talk about COVID-19 in Africa" (2020). A version of Chapter 19 was published in part in *The Nation* as "Vaccine Nationalism Is Patently Unjust" (2021) and in part in Al Jazeera as "Africa's vaccine crisis: It's not all about corruption" (2021).

This book is printed using paper from registered sustainable and managed sources.

www.hurstpublishers.com

Printed in Great Britain by Bell and Bain Ltd, Glasgow

For Lorna

CONTENTS

FOREWORD

In his 1947 novel *The Plague*, French author Albert Camus expresses the morbid mundanity of a pandemic. 'The trouble is,' Camus writes, "there is nothing less spectacular than a pestilence and, if only because they last so long, great misfortunes are monotonous".[1] More than a story about disease, Camus' fictional account of how the bubonic plague swept through a small town in French Algeria during the 1940s is a story about the fears and anxieties of human beings dealing with a collective challenge that they don't fully understand. How does it change their relationship with authority? How does it change their relationships with each other? How does it change their perception of risk and the kind of things they are willing to give up as they confront it? What are the things they are unwilling to let go of? What is it about these large-scale disasters that collides so violently with the way we think about what it means to be human, that makes us channel more energy into separating ourselves—into the contaminated and the uncontaminated—than into coming together to fight the disease?

"Pestilence is in fact very common," Camus writes, and I underline furiously, "but we find it hard to believe in a pestilence when it descends upon us."[2] I read *The Plague* while I was myself in quarantine after a positive PCR test for COVID-19. Thankfully,

FOREWORD

I was infected less than a month after receiving a booster vaccine, so my symptoms remained mild. For two years, I had managed to successfully evade the disease, first under strict self-quarantine in Nairobi, and then by building myself a travel plan based on the guidance provided by experts and the prevalence of the virus in different countries at the time. However, just when I was on the road for a Christmas vacation in December 2021, a new and highly contagious strain—Omicron—was discovered, and many protections we had previously relied upon turned out to be less effective. The hollowness of the promises about the whole world being "in this together" became truly evident when the entire African continent was branded with a scarlet letter of contagion by several countries, notably in Europe, despite the fact that COVID-19 was far more widespread there. The only thing the Botswanan and South African scientists, who discovered the Omicron variant, did was warn the world that the virus had changed—a change later found to have already been underway in Europe before it was detected in Africa. But it was enough for countries and regions to ban travel from almost all African countries.

The "after" that we had all desperately hoped was upon us after two years of lockdowns, restrictions and intense sacrifice was once again out of reach; the world was looking more and more like a place in which being black and African was enough for baseless fears of contagion.

* * *

What should a book reflecting on a pandemic be about?

When people ask me what I do, the most concise answer I can offer is that I am a storyteller. So much of what we all do in our daily lives as individuals, or as members of a community or a society, is in response to story, specifically the stories we tell ourselves about who we are. Storytellers are not just entertainment at children's parties. Storytellers are people who try to give order to the different threads of our existence. Storytellers are people who infuse our experiences with the flavour of our hopes and aspirations, simply by naming them and placing them in relation to those of others. Storytellers are people who fix history in place so that, at the very least, we can try to remember things correctly. Storytellers come in all forms, whether journalists, historians, novelists, essayists or poets. The composition might differ, but fundamentally we are all trying to do the same thing. We are trying to verbalise things that we feel need to be said, lest they be forever lost to time or memory. For me, the form of the work has always been less important than the function of the work. I am a storyteller, not just because of a particular type of work in a particular moment in history, but because I use narrative to try to make sense of the world for myself and for others.

What is the story of the pandemic about?

A moment like this, where history draws a bold line between the before and the after, is a call to action for artists and storytellers. Life invites us to do what so many are unable to do because of the way in which our societies are structured: to stop time, mark moments and invite reflection. Renowned African American author Toni Morrison once said that in times of crisis, the artists must get to work. And this pandemic, in which art emerged so ferociously as an outlet and a balm for so many, only to be neglected in the efforts to rebuild, is a moment for those who create and those who tell stories to remind us of why art matters. A book about a pandemic should not just be about the crisis; it should illuminate what the crisis meant and what the crisis could mean.

In March 2020, I was on one of the last flights from Cape Town to Nairobi before both cities were locked down due to the COVID-19 pandemic, for what turned out to be at least a year. Of course, I didn't know this at the time. Like most people, I believed the governments when they told us that we would only have to bear a few months of sacrifice to ride out the worst of the wave before we could all get back to normal. Even though we had witnessed the disease tear through Asia, then Europe, and then finally North America, somehow, four months in, Africa had been spared the worst of it. The lockdown in South Africa was announced several days after I returned to Nairobi; I cancelled a few appointments and settled into a rhythm of virtual book clubs and meet-ups with friends, while restricting my social bubble only to family. It was supposed to be three months. But four months later, listening to the eerie silence of a Nairobi without its nightlife, unsure of how work would continue, it was clear that this was not a temporary interruption. This was a seismic shift—a giant crack in the ground between the before and the after.

A book about the pandemic should be a dirge for everything we lost and a sonnet for everything good we learnt about ourselves.

In the third year of the crisis, we still find ourselves stuck between analogy and speculation, knowing that the disease has fundamentally changed our world, but not knowing when we can finally declare it over so we can begin to grapple with what "after" might look like. We know that there was some good revealed about our shared humanity, but there was also a great deal of bad. We saw generosity and selfishness at scale. We saw racism and ableism tip the scales on how the value of different lives could be measured, all in the service of this big nebulous totem we call "the Economy". We said goodbye to people we loved fiercely far too soon. We were reminded that doctors, teachers and nurses are the wheels on which our ideas of civilisation roll, only to watch those with power deny them the very basics they needed to be kept safe. We argued passionately with our friends and family about what it means to do Science. The pandemic, like all pandemics before, posed a question, asking us why we built the societies we lived in. At the start, we were promising, but by the end—or perhaps more accurately the middle, because we still don't really know how this all ends—it was clear that we were struggling with the course material.

Writing is how I make sense of the world. How do we make sense of leaders and people with power scrambling to rush us back to "normal", papering over so much suffering? How do we reconcile the need to heal and restore while holding onto the knowledge that we need to do so much better, not just return to "normal"? How do we hold on to the notion of global solidarity when powerful countries have found it so easy to leave more than two-thirds of the world behind when trying to find a way forward? The knot that has been tugging away at me as I've watched this pandemic unfold—the thing that I am desperate to make sense of—is how will we remember this properly? Partly so it doesn't happen again, but also so that we don't lose our place in the story. Fifty years from now, when someone is trying to figure out what people from different parts of the world were doing when the pandemic hit, it won't just be about the science or the medicine. It will also be about our communities and our societies, how we either pulled together or fell apart. Maybe writing it out will begin to untangle these knots.

The story about the pandemic should be a story about all of us.

I trust the virologists, researchers and doctors to ensure that we get an accurate picture of the science of the pandemic. And I'm sure medical anthropologists will eventually help us understand why we behaved the way we did. But I think back on one of the last major pandemics, when HIV/AIDS tore through my community and others around the world (and still hangs over so many of us), and I worry about what will happen if this story is not told properly. I think about how that story is remembered—all the key choices and actions that people took to survive, especially how ordinary people changed everything within their

communities to navigate the weight and devastation of that season of disease—and I worry that as we are chasing "normal", we
risk leaving some key details behind. What was so great about
"normal" anyway?

The definitive account of the COVID-19 pandemic will be
written by someone else. But it would be a loss, I think, for a
storyteller not to invite a moment of reflection. I'm telling this
story because it's important for us to agree on how we survive
these things, so we can be ready for the next one. These notes
are an opportunity to gather together stray and seemingly dis-
connected threads into some kind of narrative that expands our
understanding of the period we are living through. So much of
who we are and how we move in the world is ultimately story. It's
the stories we tell ourselves about what happened and why, what
our role was in the situation and what other people did or didn't
do that, more than anything else, influence our outlook on life.
Ugandan-British novelist Jennifer Nansubuga Makumbi has a
prize-winning short story called "Let's Tell This Story Properly".
What a powerful invitation. I think we should take her up on it.

What's the point of telling you all this? What's the point of
writing all this down? The point is to tell this story properly.
What people decide to do once they hear the story is up to them.
The storyteller only has one obligation, and that is to tell the
story properly. The essays in this collection are deliberately swift
and hopefully sharp because they are holding a space open. The
only way to eat an elephant is one bite at a time. These are small
bites that hopefully help us make sense of the big elephant of life
with, around and not-quite-after the pandemic. They are as
much for me as they are for you, the reader. As a student of
history, I know what it is to look back on the historical record
and to find a deafening silence, caused not by the absence of
information at the time, but by the failure to stop and take stock.
As an African, I know what it is to exist on the periphery of

people's imagination, to be one of the many whose histories are not deemed worth recording or retelling.

There are many reasons why the story of COVID-19 might not be told properly in the long run. Let's try and tell this story properly.

A NOTE ON TERMINOLOGY

I don't like the word "Western" or the concept of "the West". I don't like the way they casually slip into our descriptions of the world and obscure so much about the marginalisation of the global poor. I don't like the way they allow those outside their purview to be conscripted into other people's stories as minor characters instead of having agency over their own lives. It's a useless construct that corresponds neither to geography nor to politics. It's not about money, either, otherwise Singapore would be a "Western" nation. All this concept of "the West" does is create a line between "us" and "them"; for those of us who are "them", it often means that even if our story gets told, it's not told by us.

The idea of "the West" is an invention, an identity created primarily to give those who claim it space to say "we are not like them". V. Y. Mudimbe, a Congolese philosopher, writes about "the invention of Africa" as a political project to construct a bogeyman against whom "West-ness" could be defined. Palestinian-American intellectual Edward Said wrote in his 1978 book *Orientalism* that "the Orient" was a fabrication that only exists in the violent fantasies of those who wish to conquer it. A handful of nations, united by histories of imperialism, invented a list of traits and then decided that those who supposedly didn't

possess them—usually the peoples who they had subjugated—
were the "Not-Us".

This word "Western" sticks on the roof of my figurative
mouth every time I try to type it out, even though the fact of
language being a shared collective experience demands that it
show up so that people can have a sense of common reference.
But it's a sticky, molasses word that trips up my train of thought
and leaves me with clumsy formulations.

Several alternatives have been proposed in recent years.
"Developed" versus "developing" countries seems insincere when
you consider all the communities in the rural USA that are living
without clean drinking water or regular access to quality medicine. "Global South" versus "Global North" is a play on geography that leaves Australia and New Zealand in a confused position. Lately, I am charmed by "people of the global majority"
because it is statistically accurate and centres our collective sense
of geography on the experiences of the mass of the world's population, rather than those of the minority. It's a formulation that
challenges us to upend the way we read and write history: not to
begin with the minority as the default and then move to the
majority as the anomalous exception, but to reverse that tendency. It's a mouthful, but it forces us to start with those lives
through which a line of best fit can be drawn, uniting experiences across disparate geographies and giving meaning to the idea
of a global collective.

But what would be the opposite of that? What would be a
good word for all the nations that conspired to deprive the
people of the global majority of access to medicine in the middle
of a pandemic? I mulled this over repeatedly as I wrote these
essays, but I am yet to come up with an alternative, so for now I
plod on with West and Western, even though they are woefully
inadequate and so devoid of basis in contemporary realities as to
be intellectually meaningless and, indeed, insincere.

A NOTE ON TERMINOLOGY

Insincere and inadequate.

An archaic hangover from a moment when the global majority did not have enough room in the collective consciousness to tell the truth about who we are.

It's commonly said that there's a battle between the West and the East, and that Africa must pick sides. But look at this pandemic. Does that argument hold when in the direst moments Africa found itself completely abandoned, treated as fundamentally disposable by both sides? Why should Africans care about the distinction between the West and the East when neither seems to wish us well? What good does it do us to take sides if our wellbeing and that of our communities is ultimately a footnote in someone else's history? Why should we subscribe to this artificial distinction between the West and the East when the treatment we experience still leaves us oppressed, regardless of who the oppressor is?

Throughout the pandemic, I found myself contemplating the words of Ghanaian independence leader Kwame Nkrumah: "we face neither East nor West, we face forward". What does "forward" mean if we do not describe ourselves as merely incidental to other parts of the world? This, to me, is a much more productive way to have a conversation about how the people of the global majority made plans to survive a worldwide pandemic. What does a "forward" look like that keeps us protected and healthy? That's far more meaningful than engaging in debates about which oppression stings less.

I use the word "Western" in this text but, as you read it, I want you to picture me in the sense of the Kiswahili phrase, *shingo upande*, with my neck twisted awkwardly away from the page, for I cannot bear such an ultimately meaningless word.

LIFE

1

REASONING BY ANALOGY

A STORY IN THREE ACTS

Act I: In the Beginning

When COVID-19 was first declared a pandemic, there was a mad rush to find an analogy to help us prepare for whatever might be coming down the pipeline. The first of these was the "Spanish Flu", although more correctly it should be known as the Great Influenza Outbreak of 1918, seeing as Spain's defining role in the spread of the disease was just being the first country to confirm it. Much like COVID-19, Ebola, Bird Flu and numerous other illnesses, scientists think it began with a virus that somehow hopped from an animal to a human being.[1] Like COVID-19, "Spanish Flu" was also a respiratory disease that forced people to wear masks in order to avoid contamination. One of the main public health responses was to urge people to stay away from each other, and to quarantine those who had been infected.

Everything that's happened with the novel coronavirus takes me back to being a child watching people around me die of a disease that we weren't even allowed to name out loud. Sometimes we called it "hive" or "SIDS". People in Western countries reached all the way back to 1918 for an analogy, even though one of the last great pandemics is still underway—even though HIV/AIDS is still with us. Because of the political choices taken between the 1980s and the 2000s, public opinion has decided that AIDS is an African disease. The "pan" in pandemic could not possibly include Them.

It turned out to be a good thing that we were forced to revisit the influenza outbreak of 1918, because so much of what we knew about it turned out to be incomplete. People assumed that the "Spanish Flu" had come from Spain, but Spain was merely the first country to admit that something bad was underway. All other major countries had declined to acknowledge the outbreak for fear that it would cause panic or that it would distress their economies, particularly in the wake of the World War I and the expensive wars they had waged to impose colonisation in Africa. The stigma of outbreak was put upon Spain for breaking the unspoken commitment that powerful nations had to not be "it"—a habit that once again reared its ugly head with the COVID-19 outbreak.

With COVID-19, there was a push in both directions: too many people were eager to repeat the mistakes of the past, but many were also determined to do things differently. Too many people were ready to call the virus the "Wuhan Flu", even as the World Health Organization (WHO) cautioned against naming diseases after places. Former US president Donald Trump called the coronavirus the "kung flu" at a political rally; his spokesperson said it was an effort to make sure people "knew that the virus came from China", though it was more likely a new face of his well-documented prejudice against all manner of minority groups.[2] The point was to instrumentalise the disease, as if stigma could be an effective way to beat it back from US shores. Prejudice had proven to be a reliable tool in Trump's political campaigns in the

United States; here he was once again drawing from the populist playbook against a different enemy. He chose not to understand that viruses cannot be roused by hate in the same way that people can.

The efforts of the WHO and other international organisations to discourage us from naming diseases after the place where they were first found, to avoid the permanent stigma that it carries, was good and important work. Still, we had to wonder why there hadn't been similar momentum around Lassa fever, named for the town in Northern Nigeria where it was discovered, or for Ebola, named after the Ebola River in the Democratic Republic of Congo. Why is this only acceptable in Africa?

It's a weighty thing, this burden that Africans must constantly carry to avoid extending the same treatment that they have received to others. When you know how deeply something stings, you are loath to subject others to the same injury, even when they don't seem to fully understand how much it hurts. Stigma is bad. No towns or regions should have to endure it, particularly when all they are "guilty" of is telling the world that something bad has happened. What would the world look like if people extended to small African villages the same generosity they extend to wealthy countries? How do we make evading stigma something that we do for all people, everywhere? Africans don't want vengeance or reprisals. Only fairness.

There is no chance that anyone with even the faintest interest in how COVID-19 travels would not have known that the outbreak began in China. The Chinese government stumbled with the way it handled their initial response—first denying the existence of the disease, then punishing those who reported it, and then insisting that the situation was under control while the virus was spreading around the world. Today, the late whistleblower Dr Lin Wenliang is celebrated as a hero even in China for letting the world know about this novel respiratory disease, but at the time he was told to "stop making false comments" by police.[3] It's hard to imagine an African country getting away with that level of myopia, but those who have power continue to tread lightly around China for various reasons. So much of the criticism that should have been levelled against the Chinese government was instead unleashed as racist attacks against Chinese people, including those who are not even Chinese citizens, as though Chinese people were not themselves the primary victims of the state's failures. It is Chinese people who have had to endure months-long lockdowns with few resources in Shanghai. It was Chinese doctors who were arrested and penalised for raising the alarm about the new disease. But many people seem unable to separate their response to governments from their response to the people they govern.

Can't two things be true at the same time? What does a critique of a system, rooted in justice and fairness for all people—including Chinese people—look like? Can't the Chinese government be held accountable while defending Chinese people from racism? Wealthy countries must answer for their failure to prepare for the crisis that unfolded across the world, compounding errors by acting in their short-term self-interest instead of participating in a global response.

Would the world have looked different if the Chinese Government had been honest about the outbreak from the beginning? Probably. That needs to be acknowledged, because so much of what went wrong in the political response to the pandemic was rooted in an inability to say things forthrightly due to the pressure to maintain the "geopolitical balance". Powerful countries can get away with things that smaller countries cannot even contemplate. The pandemic taught us that the multipolar world, looking both East and West, is just as dangerous for poor countries as the unipolar. Justice remains an elusive aspiration when the system worships and rewards force over fairness, regardless of how many centres of power exist.

REASONING BY ANALOGY

In Kiswahili, we say *fahali wawili wakipigana, nyasi ndio huu-mia*. When two bulls fight, it is the grass that gets hurt. The wealthy countries are caught in a struggle over who deserves to be the one true hegemon or, at least, who should be the main centre of power in a multipolar world. The pandemic demonstrated how much the rest of us suffer when international relations are dictated by these fights. It is the people of the global majority who pay the price when the US president focuses more on spreading hate than participating in a coordinated global response to a virus that does not recognise nationality. When the Chinese government is more concerned with saving face than preventing catastrophe, the disease inevitably slips through the cracks. When the government of the richest country in the world is more interested in catching China in a lie than putting resources towards addressing the global or even domestic crisis, then the global crisis deepens. And the rest of us—blades of grass waving in the wind—must live with the consequences of these choices: a disease that no one was ready for and from which we don't know if we will ever fully recover.

Act II: How We Know

Two interesting and interconnected puzzles have surfaced throughout our shared experience of the pandemic. How do you know that something happened if the place where you go to find information about it does a bad job of telling the story? How do you know how something happened if the people it affected cannot agree on events? Both of these puzzles are part of the same bigger question that too few people in the world today are working to answer: what does it mean to know?

I worry a lot about how the archive of this current historical moment will tell the story of where Africans were and what they were doing when the COVID-19 pandemic struck. Misinformation has been an enormous problem throughout it. It led to people proposing all kinds of untested cures and rejecting well-documented science. It led to massive conspiracy theories about governments that are incapable of keeping electricity on or water running twenty-four hours a day suddenly developing the capacity to microchip the entire world. It led to paranoia about powerful individuals and powerful governments spreading fear to enhance their control. But this wasn't an African problem, at least not in the way that those who work regularly on misinformation thought it would. Instead, it turned out to be a major problem in individualistic societies where the concept of freedom had been distorted to mean the individual over the collective. Days of protests in Western countries over mask mandates and vaccination requirements forced governments to capitulate too early to absurd demands to end restrictions before the pandemic was truly over. The rush to return to "normal" in the West meant that children were forced to go back to full-time, in-person education before scientists could even confirm that vaccines would protect them from COVID-19.

So, why is so much of the fight against misinformation framed around the idea that if it's a bad problem over there it will be a far worse problem over here? What are we assuming that people in Africa know or cannot know when we say, "if it's bad here it must be worse there"? What are we presuming about what happens to information about illness and disease once it enters African societies?

There isn't really a single place where you can learn about how the influenza outbreak of 1918 played out in Africa. The historical record of this pandemic barely mentions the continent. In the archives of countries like Kenya and Nigeria, you can find a great deal about how the colonial administrations of the day responded, including thorough documentation of urban deaths and of the measures British authorities took to respond to the crisis. Some contemporary scientists have turned these records into essays and journal articles, and tried to draw lessons from them.[4] But you have to read these archival documents in the context within which they were produced, which isn't always the strongest suit of scientists who are merely trying to find analogies that they can use to prevent outbreaks from happening again. This historical evidence is largely from the perspective of colonial administrators, who, at the very moment of writing these documents, were engaged in a violent process of breaking down and fundamentally reorganising the societies they were writing about.

What does it mean to know something when this knowledge is framed by the anxieties, perceptions, fears and desires of people whose underlying intent is to cause harm? These are the kind of questions that people working with colonial archives are constantly battling with. There are always gaps and threads that lead to nothing, because the person who curated the archive—who decided which stories were and weren't worth preserving— wanted from the very beginning to belittle and demean the oppressed people. When we work with these kinds of archives, we always have to consider not just what the text says, but also what it doesn't say and why. Dealing with colonial archives requires an extra interpretive step, because an archive in itself is part of the project of oppression—the wilful unseeing of what the Other was doing at a given historical moment. These interpretive acts can only go so far in filling in the blanks, and humanity is collectively sentenced to lose whatever doesn't get explicitly protected.

The first colonists arrived in Kenya in the late nineteenth century; the territory was declared a protectorate of the British Crown in 1897, and the colony was consolidated in 1920. And between 1897 and 1918, there was a constant cycle of violent collision with, and resistance to, colonisation across the entire area that would eventually become the colony of Kenya. There was a raft of legislation designed to break the people's spirit, including racist prohibitions on "loitering" or "vagrancy", aimed at criminalising black urban existence and creating a pool of convict labour that could be used to turn the colony profitable (see Chapter 5). The violent introduction of taxes—such as hut taxes based on how many windows you had, as well as poll taxes—not only changed peoples' lives (for example, by literally inspiring them to build houses with fewer windows), but were also intended to create a need for money. Needing money meant that Kenyans had to work, and, at that time, the only people who provided jobs that paid in money were the colonial administrators, and perhaps a handful of Indian traders.

Some of the documents are concerned with the impact of the outbreak on labour and not the psychological experience of surviving a novel disease. They count the number of dead as those who were no longer available for work, not as humans who had lost their lives. They record death as a bureaucratic experience and not a political one; they do not capture how widespread, unexpected death could have contributed to the eventual collapse of the resistance to colonisation. They don't tell us how local people reacted to the bizarre treatment rituals prescribed by the colonial administration, or what local healers could have come up with instead. We know, for example, that the Quechua people indigenous to South America had been using quinine to treat malaria long before Spanish Jesuit priests brought the treatment back to Rome around the early seventeenth century; what did the traditional healers in Africa prescribe for the treatment of influenza in 1918? What did they do with the information about the new disease once they received it and decided that it was something that people needed to know?

I'm not interested in conversations or anxieties about superstition or religion. I am interested in how societies turn information into knowledge; different peoples, influenced by the unique ways that they organise facts, create different ways of knowing. Anyone who has ever watched the work of a herbalist—someone who believes that there is medicine in the natural world—will tell you that there is a method to it. It is often based on what mainstream philosophies of science would call inference: watching how bodies respond to various iterations of herbal mixtures and determining from that which combinations and in which doses work best. This knowledge is then passed on from generation to generation. There is a rigour to it.

What does it mean to know something when the contexts in which the paths to knowledge are created are so different? This is the key question we all need to answer if we are to get to the heart of why so many people from so many backgrounds were ready to disbelieve information they received about the pandemic. This was predominantly a problem of individualistic societies in the global minority—of people who were determined not to be told what to do by their governments. Is this cul de sac where individualism will end up?

We talk about misinformation and disinformation as if they have no precedent, as if we have always agreed on what it means to know. But I think we are experiencing a fundamental disconnect between an approach that insists knowing is an individual experience, and one that stresses the role of the collective in developing knowledge together. This is why I am curious about how African societies processed the influenza outbreak: how did peoples with different cultures of knowledge production receive that information and then decide what to do with it? We have lost and continue to lose entire knowledge systems, and many people want some version of them back. They want to return to ways of knowing that are rooted in their communities, rather than descending from a secret place on high.

There is a false dichotomy between the idea of starting in nature for solutions and a belief in science to develop those solutions, particularly because so much of what we consume as medicine is derived from plants. Andry Rajoelina, President of Madagascar, and John Pombe Magufuli, former president of Tanzania, relied entirely on unproven herbal remedies as a response to COVID-19. They advocated for herbal treatments like Covid-Organics, an untested Artemisia-based drink developed in Madagascar early in the pandemic, which was soon exported to Tanzania.[5] The problem, to me, wasn't so much that they sought a solution in nature, but that they encouraged the use of a putative cure without checking if it worked. The efficacy of this treatment was tested on only around twenty people over a matter of three weeks. What kind of inference can you generate in such a short amount of time? They put their entire populations at great risk because of this false binary, this unwillingness to even engage with the science. The result was effectively a massive clinical trial on poor people in both their countries, without any kind of oversight. There's a reason why medical testing protocols exist; evading them in the name of seeking a solution in nature is not the answer. We should be able to see why the rigorous methods of science are necessary, and why they offer answers, without being entirely dismissive of the entire idea of looking to nature.

What would further investigation into the inferential knowledge of African indigenous people about the 1918 influenza outbreak have yielded? What would we have known that we don't currently because the people who documented their experiences were not interested in the human aspects of the novel virus? This is the loss I mourn: the clues that traditional healers confronted with this new disease might have found about how to handle it. The ways of thinking that are displaced by a monochrome version of the world. Different ways of ordering questions and different sources of solutions. We'll never really know what those traditional healers may have unearthed which could have informed our understanding about the challenge we face now. How do we articulate that without being interpreted as "anti-science"?

The debates about science and the pandemic have made it very difficult to have these kinds of conversations in public. There is an alarming contingent of people who have become fundamentalist in both their belief and disbelief in science. Any suggestion that the Scientific Method, rooted in Western philosophy, may not be the only way to generate knowledge is met with derision, and usually dismissed. But it is equally, if not more, alarming how many people are ready to disbelieve science altogether, as if all methods of discernment are invalid. As if knowledge itself is an undesirable thing. On the one hand, we are told that we are superstitious, crazy and wrong, even if all we are saying is, "what if there are other places to look for the answers that we might need?" But on the other, even as I write this, there are still far too many people in all corners of the world who are convinced that COVID-19 is a political conspiracy, even as we tell them about the loved ones we have lost or of the bodies that are still battling to recover months after infection.

There are too many people who still dismiss the science of vaccines, as if vaccines had not done the bulk of the heavy-lifting needed to change the course of history. Polio, measles, tuberculosis and diphtheria are diseases that less than a century ago killed people painfully and in alarming numbers, but today we can hardly pronounce their names. All banished from mainstream consciousness by vaccines. And it isn't just random people angrily tweeting from the darkness of their mothers' basements who hold anti-vax beliefs. Back and forth, back and forth, back and forth. What if there are clues elsewhere beyond the world of patents, trade secrets and gatekeepers? What tools and methods could we use to uncover those clues and see where they lead us? What would examining them fairly help us learn about ourselves?

The chairman of an independent organisation known as the Kenya Catholic Doctors Association—unaffiliated with either the Catholic Church or mainstream doctors' groups—famously declared in March 2021 that COVID-19 vaccines were unnecessary, before succumbing to the virus himself just weeks later.[6] But this culture of disbelief is not an "African" problem. If anything, it has turned out to be worse in more developed countries where more people depend on the Internet to get their daily news and information. In Kenya, on the other hand, those fighting against disinformation worked with community-driven ways of knowing to stop it becoming widespread. People came together to translate health advice into local languages. Barazas, or informal meetings in villages and towns, were called so that people with authority could speak directly to the community about the new disease. Radio stations invited guests to call in and ask medical professionals questions. Combatting disinformation was not an individual experience—the argument was never that the individual should simply know better. It was a community experience guided by cultures of care: we all need to work together to survive this.

In the US, social media has emerged as a site for creating and sharing misinformation about the pandemic at alarming speed, dissuading people from getting vaccinated and ultimately feeding into the staggering death toll that keeps on climbing.[7] In countries where people are still dependent on traditional media for their information, this momentum has been somewhat disrupted because of institutional guardrails like professional codes of conduct or media ethics. It's no small irony that the strongest impetus for disbelieving the science about vaccines is in societies from which many of the philosophies that shape this science are rooted. Indeed, it's probably an indicator of a social phenomenon that is located elsewhere, perhaps that the increasing commercialisation of health and science has fuelled a general mistrust of those who manufacture medicine. If the separation of Church and State saved democracy, can the separation of medicine and profit save us from the anti-scientists?

These new cultures of knowing are also part of the story of technology. Technology has not only changed the way we share and receive information. It has also changed the way we believe. It has brought so much knowledge closer to the people, and this is a good thing. But we have been slow to adapt our ways of processing this information. The individualistic philosophies of knowledge that encourage the intrepid explorer to go off and collect information and process it merely by his or her own creativity and enterprise is reaching its limits in the digital age. The idealised scientist of this approach is a lone worrier and warrior, plugging away at a single question that will answer at least one of the great questions of civilisation. We teach people that the point of science is individual discovery instead of a process of deepening and broadening our collective experience of living and being. We celebrate discovery and not collaborative investigation. We forget that we aren't universally grounded in the same philosophies of what it means to know.

More importantly, we don't know how to talk to each other across these differences. We are often arrogant and condescending, or abrasive and defensive—fundamentalist—when we should be humble in the face of what we might not know even as we grow in knowledge. We assume that everyone receives and processes information as an individual and therefore that merely giving people the correct information is enough. But we are learning that for the vast majority of people, knowing is a collective effort. Knowing means conversations with people that we trust for various reasons—not just because they are scientists who have endured the lonely work of seeking knowledge, but because they are people we know or people who have a platform.

We still don't really understand how to process this new experience of how people come to know and believe, and that is perhaps why three years and millions of deaths later, we still have people with incredibly large platforms who can manipulate seemingly intelligent people into rejecting reality in favour of a story that makes them feel good. We have made important efforts to change the quality and quantity of information that people receive. But we need more investigation into the different ways of knowing—how the people who exist outside institution-alised science come to understand information, process facts and then modify their behaviour in light of it. Knowledge is as much about trust and belief as it is about information. We're doing a lot of work on information. But we need to learn more about how people come to trust and believe.

This is why the way African scientists processed the arrival of the 1918 influenza interests me. We know that outside the Western philosophical tradition, knowing is a much more collec-tive enterprise. I'm curious about how knowledge of things yet unexperienced is processed in contexts where to know and to believe is collaborative. I'm curious about the pathways through which facts are generated and then transmitted, the ways they go from novel information to established belief, because I think this reveals volumes about the way the Internet is changing what it means to know.

Act III: How We Move

Renowned French-Martinican philosopher Frantz Fanon wrote in his seminal essay "Concerning Violence" that "The settler makes history and is conscious of making it. ... [But] the history which he writes is not the history of the country which he plun-ders but the history of his own nation in regard to all that she skims off, all that she violates and starves."[8] The histories of colonised nations as catalogued by colonial archives are not designed to be true: they are designed to preserve power.

The 1918 influenza pandemic came at the tail end of the process of consolidating the British Empire's hold on the country that would become Kenya. The racism that would characterise how the colony was governed was being bureaucratised and formalised. To be honest, I'm surprised that they even counted our dead, although it's fascinating how the cruellest systems in the world always make an effort to document the widespread killing as part of the process of sanitising it. The apartheid government of South Africa kept meticulous records. As did the Nazi regime in Germany. As did most colonial authorities around the world. The logic seems to be if they carefully chronicled the number of people they tortured and murdered, then the killing itself could not have been unjust. As long as the records show that it was done to the standards the bureaucracy demands, then the actual idea of ending lives for no reason and at devastating scale is more palatable to the system in which it occurs.

The stories of how ordinary people adapted to the new reality of the 1918 pandemic—fundamentally, how we survived—are mired in this politics. We know a lot about what the colonial administration did: the quarantines, the cessation of movements, the pseudo-remedies such as forcing people to gargle potassium permanganate or take a teaspoon of paraffin oil. We know less about the choices that people had to make every day. What is the Kiswahili or Ekegusii word for influenza? Does it distinguish between the flu and a cold? How did people warn each other? What accommodations did they make in their home life? We know a little more about what happened in Nigeria, and Lagos specifically, because it was the largest port in the region.[9] There was also more of an effort to listen to African health practitioners who were otherwise excluded from the healthcare service in the colony because they were black.[10]

Transport systems were a big part of how influenza moved around the world. In Kenya, a lot of its spread was attributed to the railway. (A key reason the British colonised this territory in the first place was to link the neighbouring, landlocked protectorate of Uganda to the coast, via Kenya.) The outbreak began in the port city of Mombasa, where conscript soldiers returning from service in the armies of various European powers are suspected to have unwittingly carried the disease back with them. Slowly it snaked its way inward along the railway line—the main transport artery in the emerging country. As the disease took hold in the coastal cities and strict containment measures began to bite, many soldiers travelled into the hinterland to return to their families. And this is how the influenza found its way across the territory in 1918.

I thought about this a lot as I endured the lockdown in Nairobi. There was a moment when many people were convinced that Africa would not be touched at all. It really looked like the virus was a Western musician on world tour, stopping on every continent except ours. The first cases in China were officially confirmed in December 2019, but even according to Chinese government records, the first cases were actually detected in November that year—but that information was deliberately suppressed.[11] Europe's first cases were reported in January 2020, and a wave of strict lockdowns soon followed there. After that came North and South America, and, by this time, the disease already had a foothold in the rest of Asia; but aside from South Africa and Egypt, much of the African continent did not record a single case until April.

By April, comparable countries outside of Africa were suffering intensely. The politics of post-coloniality almost mandate that Anglophone countries compare themselves to each other. When searching for comparisons to predict what might happen in Anglophone Africa, most people looked to India, Malaysia or other former British colonies. One important step towards decolonising public health would be to break out of the lines that imperialism drew and to start comparing like to like. The population of India is equal to, if not slightly larger, than the population of all of Africa. I've always found it to be a facile and lazy comparison.

It is important for our gaze to travel elsewhere even when our bodies cannot. It is important to see the world beyond the lines that history has drawn across our lives. I looked to similar countries with similar problems to try to get a sense of what might be coming for us. Kenya and Ecuador, for example, are both on the equator, with high-altitude capital cities and low, coastal second cities. Both have a deeply unequal population and major informal settlements in their urban areas. Politics in both has been tumultuous over the last twenty years, resulting in the rapid devaluation of the Kenyan shilling and Ecuador's decision to officially use the US dollar as its currency.

COVID-19 devastated Ecuador. A wave of students coming back from Spain and Italy after the lockdowns there brought the disease to the small country. Most of the country's early cases were in Guayaquil, officially the second city but in fact larger than the capital Quito by some calculations. At its worst, so many people were dying in this city that morgues were overwhelmed, and people left bodies in the street for the authorities to find.[12] The health system became saturated in a matter of weeks, and people who suffered from other diseases struggled to find reasonable care.[13] Many of those who died lived in informal settlements. Even the crematorium could not burn the bodies fast enough. Ecuador ranked eighty-sixth in the latest Human Development Index: Kenya ranked 143rd.[14] On paper, at least, if a similar situation unfolded in Kenya, it would be an unmitigated disaster, and there was reason to be concerned.

By the time of publication, that situation has not unfolded. I don't think it's because Kenyans are miraculously immune to COVID-19, even though I trust scientists who say that youth is a significant factor in improving collective experience of the disease. It makes sense that the youngest continent in the world would have the lowest rates of coronavirus; young people are less likely to experience serious illness, and serious illness is known to accelerate the spread of the disease.

Africa is also the least-connected continent in the world. Roughly 100,000 flights take off and land every day globally, and the smallest share of these occur in the world's second-largest continent.[15] The most-connected countries—South Africa and Egypt—had the worst outbreaks in the first wave. During the window when COVID-19 was primarily being spread by travel, Africa simply had the least exposure, and by the time the disease did land, we had already witnessed the devastation that it caused elsewhere and had had more time to prepare. People underestimate how crucial human action is in situations like this. In Kenya, for example, we had our first lockdown at an earlier point in the pandemic than Ecuador; it was a more complete lockdown; and there was a faster and more complete mask mandate. There was no extended period of debating masks, and that slowed down the contagion considerably. If anything, the situation in Africa should be telling the world what COVID-19 could have looked like if universal measures were put in place quicker. Kenya's decision to sever the transport links and stop people from travelling into and out of the country seems to have slowed the spread of the disease, even though it caused other forms of widespread harm.

Transport changed dramatically during the pandemic, although it seems that these changes will not be permanent. There was significant resistance to keeping restrictions or policies in place even a second longer than they are absolutely required, leading many countries to end them much earlier than experts recommended. Is wearing a mask really that much of an inconvenience in the face of a devastating disease? The UK ended its restrictions on masking on airplanes in March 2022, celebrating the occasion with triumphant promotional videos from cabin crew in full uniform.[16] Three weeks later, in April, airlines in the country were cancelling flights en masse because too many staff members were off sick with COVID-19.[17] The same pattern played out across other European airports, with unexpected delays and slowdowns in Amsterdam, Brussels, Dublin, Frankfurt and many more. Airlines argued that they were understaffed because travel resumed so quickly that they didn't have a chance to rehire all the staff that had been laid off due to the pandemic.

But what this betrays is a rush to return to "normal" before the lessons of the pandemic had been learnt. Returning to "normal" meant European tourists travelling around the world for their spring holidays, even while cases there continued to trend upwards. It meant Westerners travelling around the world as if nothing at all had happened, even though many countries were and are still struggling to vaccinate their populations. It meant people continuing to bring illness into places that were not well set up to deal with it. Despite the experiences of that first wave, the lesson remained unlearnt. What does it say about the "normal" we have built if it cannot stop to attend to life? As the hubs for global travel, international solidarity would perhaps require some of these countries to contemplate their obligations to other nations in thinking about the measures that need to remain in place. Instead, they have capitulated to the anxieties of people who refuse to sacrifice their comfort for the greater good.

On a flight to New York in April 2022, a member of the cabin crew of the US airline came to my seat where I was wearing a triple layer mask and told me, "you know you don't have to wear the mask any more". As if keeping the mask on as the pandemic raged was the irrational choice. Other travellers have made the same observation, because it really jumps out at you at the airport. There is an irony in having to take your shoes off and essentially present yourself naked in front of a security scanner because one person tried and failed to detonate a shoe bomb more than twenty years ago, versus being encouraged to be lax in the face of a pandemic that has killed at least 6.3 million people worldwide in less than three calendar years. No one is asking for permanent. But can we not at least wait until the emergency is over before rushing back to "normal"?

2

LOCKDOWN

Lockdown was the 2020 word of the year for the Collins English Dictionary. In some countries, it evoked memories of applauding healthcare workers on the balconies at 7 p.m. In others, it meant unprovoked arrests and beatings from police officers simply for the crime of existing in the wrong place at the wrong time. Some people used the time to learn how to make banana bread, just out of curiosity. Others learnt how to survive on next to nothing as jobs disappeared and government support failed to materialise. For some, it was the only thing of significance that happened in 2020; for others, it was the most significant thing that didn't happen, or didn't happen fast enough. Single people in large cities confronted the realities of modern loneliness, which could not be healed merely through social media. Families buckled under the strain of forced intimacy. In the same cities that some people merrily tweeted their way through the pandemic, uninsured, underpaid and overworked food delivery drivers took on inexplicable risk to keep them fed and happy in that new reality. A word that should have said something about the pandemic as a global experience instead was testimony to how divided and differentiated the world really is.

Lockdowns continued perhaps in their most extreme iteration even well into 2022, in cities like Shanghai. They were supposed to be temporary—just a few weeks to allow healthcare systems to catch up with the overwhelming demands. They were an act of solidarity. We clapped for healthcare workers at the same time every day just to let them know that we were standing with them. Everything that could go virtual did, and everything that could not stopped. For the most part. Eventually we found out that the rules in almost all countries were elastic when powerful people were involved, but that didn't really matter at the time. We believed that we were all in it together, that we all needed to make sacrifices in order to get through it.

The idea of locking down a city to save people from disease is not in itself new, so there's no need to frame 2020 as unprecedented in history. Medical historian Eugenia Tognotti published an excellent paper in 2013 that looked at the history of quarantine in Western Europe, beginning with the bubonic plague of around 1347–52 and ending with the influenza outbreak of 1918.[1] In many ways, the article is a reminder that regardless of our notions of history, human behaviour remains remarkably repetitive. Our ideas of how to confront the threat of death at scale are still nearly identical to how Venetians of the fourteenth century treated those who suffered from the plague: isolate them from the general population and wait for the disease to pass. Quarantining sick people was also common in other societies that have had to deal with highly contagious illnesses, like leprosy, for example.

One major difference between 2020 and fourteenth-century Europe is the sheer numbers of us calling cities home, meaning that a lockdown isn't simply a process of isolating several dozen people from the rest of the village, but trying to control and interfere with the movement of millions of people. The 2014–16 Ebola outbreak was perhaps the first time that today's generation saw governments of all types try to pass rules to say that movement into or out of certain towns, cities or countries was prohibited. It often failed, for various reasons, not least of which was that governments usually didn't give the healthy people caught up in those lockdowns a chance to find other ways of making life meaningful, including by providing basic necessities. International lockdown orders during the Ebola epidemic were often racist and were punitive against the entire continent, even when the outbreak was localised. People get scared and anxious when they don't have enough information, and being told that you are facing a highly contagious and dangerous disease while being unable to move took its toll on many people, some who simply tried to escape. In 2020, this pattern was repeated in many countries where lockdown rules were poorly explained: people tried to find a way around them and ended up spreading the disease.

I spent my lockdown in Nairobi and saw my hometown in a way that I had never seen it before. Nairobi is not a twenty-four-hour city, at least not in the way that people who make urban policy use the phrase. When the Uhuru Kenyatta administration came to power in 2013, it promised to make the capital a twenty-four-hour city, meaning a big metropolis where you could still find somewhere open to get food or drink after you had been out dancing with your friends until 4 a.m. But the security challenges that the city faces have made this dream unattainable. At most, Nairobi is probably a twenty-hour city, in which early birds and night owls trade shifts and drowsily peer over at each other in the rush-hour traffic. It's a city that comes alive at around 4:30 a.m. when the food delivery trucks from the countryside roll in, and descends into a muted hum at around midnight when the indoor bars and clubs really start to take off. It's not that there aren't people out and about between midnight and 4:30 a.m. It's just that they're not engaged in the kind of businesses that the government wants to use in their promotional materials. People still party, but several years ago we got into the habit of staying out all night instead of trying to make it back home after a certain time. Between the drunk drivers and the car jackers, it just made more sense to stay where you were until the sun came up.

Yet every sunset from late March to July 2020, lockdown shrouded Nairobi in a silence that was dramatic and chilling, nothing at all like the city we all knew. On 27 March 2020, a dawn-to-dusk curfew was imposed across Kenya. On 6 April, the government announced what they called a cessation of movement, which is an elaborate spoonful of sugar designed to stamp official-dom onto the process. The initial three-week ban on movement eventually extended to three and a half months, within which travel into and out of the four worst-affected counties—Nairobi, Mombasa, Kilifi and Kwale—was strictly prohibited.

The ban on movement had a terrible impact on so many people around the country. It meant that children who were in boarding schools were not allowed to go home to visit their parents over the Easter break, extending their time away from their family to almost seven months. It meant that people who lived in one county and worked in another—particularly common between the capital and the surrounding areas—could not get to work. Long-haul transport slowed to a devastating crawl, holding up supplies to nearby landlocked countries. The lockdown was also summarily announced, and the rules kept changing. As with anywhere in the world where middle- and upper-class people can be found, they panic-bought toilet paper, pulses and legumes. But for the vast majority of city residents who live from day to day, even the two- or three-month horizon was a great deal to ask.

I should say that, in principle, I'm not opposed to lockdowns as a public health measure. I understand the thinking behind them. A basic tenet of living in a society is that, at some point, we have to concede some rights for the greater good. But these concessions must be freely given and not coerced; they must be the best or only way to achieve this greater good; and we must be able to claw back our rights when the emergency period passes. The major problem with the lockdowns in much of the world was that concessions were taken by force rather than given; that police interpreted their role as beating civilians until the virus left our collective bodies; that communication with people fell apart quickly; that people who had power and money opted out almost as soon as restrictions were in place; and, most importantly, that not enough was done to protect vulnerable people from the secondary impact of these measures. The lockdowns intensified the injustices that many in our societies were already living with.

Millions of people lost their jobs and their livelihoods because of COVID-19 restrictions and, in many countries, large companies got more relief and financing from the state than the poorest of the poor, translating into growing profits and soaring executive pay, while poverty grew. During lockdowns in India, migrant labourers got stuck in Delhi with no job, no way home and with poor-quality aid.[2] Some Kenyans in Nairobi did get financial help through partnerships between development agencies, foreign embassies and local mobile phone companies.[3] But the real superstars in many countries were the neighbourhood associations and community groups that came together to protect people from loneliness and hunger. Mutual aid groups in Nairobi and other urban centres figured out how to get help while large companies were still building the architecture of their response. It was a small win in a sea of devastating loss: discovering once again that thread of community.

These lockdowns were not equal things. I was one of the people who was initially opposed to a travel ban because they were and still are applied so selectively. When the virus mutated into the Omicron strain in November 2021, I was caught in the cross-fires, stuck overseas for two weeks because I live in an African country. In the grand scheme of things, I was alright—it was a temporary setback rather than a permanent loss. But this wasn't the case for people who were subsequently prevented from seeing their families, for example, and it certainly doesn't diminish the violence that underpins the unequal way the lockdowns against Africans were imposed. Botswanan and South African scientists who had been religious in their genomic sequencing alerted the world to the fact that the virus had changed.[4] For their efforts, they were rewarded with a movement ban; some countries went so far as to ban travel from the entirety of Africa, as if it were not the second most populous continent on the planet.

Soon enough, it became clear that what the Botswanans and South Africans had done was to tell the world about a variant that was already running rampant in Europe. Yet few travel bans were instituted against European countries, even while individual nations within that continent continued to report rapidly increasing cases. Meanwhile, the damage was done, and the prejudice was already visible. The November–December 2021 lockdowns reflected a world primed to disbelieve African scientists, itching to ban African people, and unwilling to listen to reason. They affirmed what we had suspected to be true: a pernicious racism underlies the way travel and mobility is managed in wealthy countries. Once wealthier countries were done hoarding medicine and saving themselves, they would find ways to lock up the rest of us, and Africans in particular, counting down the days until COVID-19 could truly become an African disease.

The principles of lockdowns and shutdowns don't hold when these measures are only applied against the Other. It's not a lockdown if beliefs about where illness and contagion reside are merely a reflection of the preoccupations of power. When we believe that disease is natural in some parts of the world and inherently unnatural in others, we betray our own bias and unjust politics. When the contours of these lockdowns matched the contours of power's prejudices—white people who believe that diseases only come from black or brown countries, rich nations who believe that viruses only belong to poor nations—then we are no longer practicing public health. We are doing something sinister.

The loss of movement was difficult for everyone, but the extent to which different people were able to find solace within these lockdowns said a lot about how deeply unequal the world is right now—and how it has gotten so much worse for billions of people. Some of us got the luxury of spending the time listening into Instagram dance parties; some people lost everything and spent much of the lockdown looking at their starving children without any idea how they would keep them alive. Of course, it would be churlish to dismiss the coping mechanisms we needed to survive the changing circumstances. Weekly Zoom quiz nights turned out to be a crucial way to maintain connections as I was separated from my family and friends by the lockdown. The point is not to pour cold water on people who reached for whatever was available to them to survive.

The point is that, centuries after the first quarantines and lockdowns were put in place to combat the Black Death, we have somehow gotten worse at providing the tools that the most vulnerable among us need to survive. The point is that, on a national and international scale, we are still be stuck in the same cycle of denying crucial help to people and then punishing them for suffering. The point is that too much of what is passed around as policy is actually a bureaucratised articulation of racist, ableist and generally exclusionary biases that are chomping at the bit, always waiting to be unleashed. The point is that, while lockdowns started out as an opportunity to demonstrate solidarity and a different way of organising our societies, they quickly disintegrated because of decisions made by those who wield power. The point is that we should have done better. We could be doing better. Lockdowns, at the very least, could have been an opportunity to reset. Instead, old vices found new expression and old violence found new reasons to be unleashed, compounding the tragedy and the harm.

3

MASKING

In June 2020, the World Health Organization quietly changed its advice on masks, recommending their use by the general public for the first time.[1] Prior to this, it had maintained that masks were unnecessary, even unhelpful, because they did not effectively protect the user from the coronavirus. It had argued that because ordinary people were not properly trained in wearing surgical or N-95 masks, the risks of cross-contamination were high. People could mishandle the masks when wearing or taking them off and rub germs into their skin; they could take them off to take a call and put them back on improperly. The WHO had also been concerned that masks would lead to a false sense of security in the wearer, who would then stop being vigilant in other simple areas—like washing their hands or avoiding close contact with others. More importantly, the WHO had contended that high demand for masks was leading to a shortage for frontline health workers around the world. "Just wash your hands and socially distance," they had advised.

Yet, by the time the WHO issued its revised guidance, masks were everywhere. Residents of Asian countries like Hong Kong and Taiwan, who had recently navigated outbreaks of respiratory illnesses like SARS and MERS, almost instinctively put on masks despite the WHO advice. In Kenya, masks became mandatory in public spaces in April 2020 (and are still required in enclosed public areas at the time of writing), and those found without one face significant fines or even arrest. In the US, while the mask was embroiled in an embedded politics of absolute, unfettered freedom, there was also a campaign to raise public awareness of the importance of community participation for making health interventions work: some states and businesses made masks mandatory; some users refused them as a violation of their personal freedom. Given a choice between liberty or death, some in the US ask, why not both?

The mask was the definitive marker of the break between the world before COVID-19 and the world after it. Its physicality was a raw symbol that something important had fractured, and its ubiquity a reminder that there was no going back anytime soon. Before January 2020, the average person would be hard-pressed to distinguish between an N-95 and a surgical mask; now we have all become entry-level experts, not just in the differences in design, but in the global supply system of these tiny rectangles with elastic loops that were increasingly framed as the only barrier between us and near-certain mass death. There were those who were religious about wearing and keeping their masks on, and there were the lazy among us who used them to protect our chins and foreheads instead of our noses and mouths. There were mask-truthers and mask-deniers: those who believed the official guidance and those who thought it was an overreaction to "just another flu".

The mask was the unofficial mascot of 2020.

As one of the people who followed WHO guidelines closely, I felt a certain sense of betrayal both in the way the organisation backtracked on their original recommendations and in the realisation that their earlier advice was not grounded entirely in science. In April 2020, renowned medical journal *The Lancet* had directly contradicted the WHO's then guidance and affirmed that masks do work, and subsequent research has shown that not only are surgical and N-95 masks effective, but so too are the cloth masks that many societies around the world have been making as shortages of clinical-standard masks bite—albeit providing a lower level of protection.[2]

All masks are not created equal, and since they were made mandatory around the world, there has been a proliferation of styles and designs. For a long time, the WHO insisted that COVID-19 is a relatively large virus that exists in droplets—i.e., in saliva or snot, but also in fine moisture that all people project when they speak or sing. The point of the mask therefore, was to stop these droplets from landing on other people's skin or on surfaces where the virus could live for an extended period of time. But two years after the start of the pandemic, the WHO finally conceded that COVID-19 is airborne, and that it wasn't enough to just stop droplets from landing: we needed masks that stopped the virus from travelling between people in the air that they breathe.[3] It was a reminder that large bureaucracies can be too slow to adapt during emergencies and this can have serious ramifications.

From a design perspective, the safest mask is the N-95 mask, which, according to the US Centers for Disease Control and Prevention (CDC), is designed to have a very close facial fit and to allow the filtration of tiny particles by forming a seal around the mouth. These are the single-use masks that surgeons wear, but you may also see them on construction sites, where they stop workers from inhaling fine powders in toxic quantities. Next step down are the surgical masks, loose fitting and held behind the ears using either two elastic bands or tied. They are also designed to be used once in medical procedures and have varying thicknesses depending on the context in which they are supposed to be used. Some masks may look like surgical masks but actually aren't, because they stop large droplets but do not filter the finest particles that can contaminate a surgical setting. They cannot protect you from diseases that are truly airborne like measles or tuberculosis, but they can stop you from touching your face if your hands are contaminated or from coughing out contagious droplets if you are ill.

Many of the cloth masks available for sale are made from cotton fabrics, which have large spaces between the individual fibres. This is precisely what makes cotton so desirable—cotton breathes. Unlike surgical or N-95 masks, which are unpleasant even for medical professionals, the breathiness of cotton reduces the likelihood that people will take them off or interfere with them just because they are uncomfortable. But it doesn't form that seal around the nose and mouth that an N-95 or even a high-quality surgical mask would, to protect you from all germs. Simply draping a bandana over your nose will protect you from say, someone's cough, but it won't protect you from measles, nor will it be effective if you touch a contaminated surface and then use that hand to scratch your nose, nor if you are continuously exposed to someone who is sick, such as if you are nursing a coronavirus patient.

Thankfully, there is a design solution that starts to resolve this problem. In Kenya and many other African countries, tailors and fashion designers experimented with open-source designs for making cloth masks safer. The CDC argues that a loose-fitting cloth mask may not effectively protect the wearer from being contaminated, but it does reduce the likelihood of the wearer contaminating others, and considering that a significant number of those who have the coronavirus have no symptoms, this can help slow down the spread of the disease.[4] Adding a filter between the layers of a two-ply cotton mask—like a tissue paper or kitchen towel—makes the mask even more effective in unpredictable situations where the wearer may be inadvertently exposed, like in a line at the bank.

By the time the Kenyan government declared a national lockdown in late March 2020, Kenyan designers, coordinated by the Kenya Fashion Council and the National Tailors' Association, were already refining this open-source design. Millions of mechanical and electronic sewing machines across the country whirred to life as scrap material and bolts of otherwise unusable fabric were turned into something meaningful. The speed at which it happened was breath-taking—the lockdown came into force on 27 March, and within days, social entrepreneur Florence Kamaitha had sets of three masks available for sale at US $5. While the government was still negotiating with export processing zones on the technicalities of shifting production to surgical masks, tailors were already distributing products within their communities. On 4 April, the government made masks mandatory in public spaces and by the middle of the following week, I was holding my own handmade, two-ply mask with a slot in the middle for a filter, from Ann McCreath and the team at KikoRomeo.

By the end of April, all major fashion designers in the country were making masks as an extension of their previous business model, for example from canvas at luggage designer Sandstorm, or dainty lace and silk affairs from bridal atelier Ogake Mosomi. And they were not simply functional, either. Most are made from the highly popular *kitenge* fabric, and masks in Nairobi became an extension of the wearer's fashion sensibilities. Some designers made masks and headwraps or bags as matching sets. Vivo Activewear included a matching scarf in its clothing collection. Peperuka branded theirs with the slogan "wacha hii korona iishe" meaning "let this Corona pass", a sly dig at the excuse that some Nairobians had been using to postpone all kinds of obligations.

More importantly, across Kenya's informal settlements, tailors quickly moved to distribute masks for free to their neighbours in tightly packed houses where social-distancing is simply impossible. Fashion designer David Avidu was featured on television in April 2020 as one of the earliest pioneers of this practice, but community benefit organisations like African Masks and SHOFCO also incorporated mask distribution into their work.[5] KikoRomeo ran a programme where the profit from each mask sold was ploughed back into a pool to allow tailors sewing masks to distribute them for free.

This response was partly prompted by the government's decision to make not wearing a mask a criminal rather than a civil offence. Kenya has a long history of police brutality and violence in slums, and tailors and community groups correctly feared that if they did not make masks available to the public quickly, the police would disproportionately punish poor residents of informal settlements with arrest and even extra-judicial execution. Their fears were borne out soon after the laws were announced: in April 2020, activist Boniface Mwangi released a video showing Kenyan police violently rounding up young men in the Korogocho slum who were wearing masks improperly (under the chin rather than on the face and nose), even though the plain clothes officers themselves were not correctly wearing them.[6]

In fact, in Kenya, like in other societies, the shape and form of mask usage is contoured by underlying dynamics that preceded the pandemic. There was public resistance to the criminalisation of non-compliance with mask mandates, but not to mask-wearing per se, in part because we are a society that has survived other widespread disease outbreaks and have had to adapt our behaviour accordingly. For African millennials like myself who are part of the roughly three-quarters of Kenya's population that is below the age of thirty-five, our defining generational marker is not avocado toast or home ownership. We are the HIV/AIDS generation that destigmatised and adapted to the omnipresence of that disease. We are the first generation for whom sex without condoms was ever an option, even sometimes with the person you are married to. We are the generation that had to get comfortable with people coming into our classrooms with wooden penises to demonstrate condom use, or who saw the purple and yellow billboards for Voluntary Counselling and Testing for HIV/AIDS proliferate on every street corner in our hometowns. Once you have re-organised your whole life around the threat and presence of HIV/AIDS, putting on a mask is not something worth fighting about.

Moreover, the rapid uptake of reusable masks in Kenya compared to countries like the UK and the US can be directly connected to its culture of reuse and recycling. Yes, Kenya has a trash problem, but if you go beyond the structural challenges of municipal waste management, you find that poor people and poor countries are the best at reusing and recycling materials; wasting things is an expensive habit that few can afford. Kenya's textile industry has struggled because of the popularity of *mitumba*—second-hand clothing dumped in Africa from Western countries—but tailors are a dime a dozen on every street owing to the demand for bespoke clothing for special occasions and the culture of repairing damaged items rather than throwing them away. Kenya's environmental street cred has been solid, and this made the pivot to reusable masks organic. In 2017, the government had also announced a nationwide ban on plastic bags, fuelling demand for reusable tote bags and baskets, including those made from cotton. For bag designers like Vintara Collections, moving from totes to masks was a no-brainer.

None of this is to say that there was 100 per cent compliance with mask-wearing. The inadequate visual messaging by the state on the seriousness of COVID-19 did a lot of damage to public consciousness. By refusing to wear masks in their own meetings and press conferences, the government sent mixed messages to citizens, causing many people to believe that they could continue to perch their masks precariously on their foreheads or under their chins, at least until they spotted a police van. Even the police, while arresting people for not wearing masks, were rarely seen wearing masks. The class dynamics of who gets away with a warning and who spends the weekend in jail—or even dies—for breaking mask regulations are stark and depressing.

But at the very least, the creativity and Kenyan twist that designers put on the mask meant that people accepted them with less resistance. We didn't waste time arguing about wearing them, and this may have been one of the tools that gave poor societies like ours some hope of navigating the realities of COVID-19. If masks were the new normal, at the very least Kenyans would look good wearing them.

4

UNMASKING

A very interesting thing happened in the US, where simply asking people to wear masks in order to curb the spread of the deadly coronavirus turned into a hot debate about personal freedom. There was chilling footage from late June 2020 of voters in a Florida county testifying before their local council on how making masks mandatory in public places was not just an affront to their personal freedom, but antithetical to the entire founding premise of the country. It didn't matter that none of what they were saying was based on fact—they were adamant and loud, which in the current US political climate doubles up as justification. And the debate about the mask mandate went all the way to top of government, with then president Donald Trump routinely refusing to wear a mask even in situations where it was required, leading in one case to a factory producing medical swabs for coronavirus testing being forced to throw out their entire daily inventory following a visit by the unmasked POTUS.[1]

Kenya, like many other African countries, made masks in public mandatory early on in the pandemic, but unlike the US, there was no debate about personal freedoms, only about the behaviour of the police. In the first nine weeks of lockdown in Kenya, the police killed fifteen people in extra-judicial executions while ostensibly enforcing government cessation of movement directives, so adding another layer of law and regulation to the public health situation.[2] The country has a history of disproportionately violent policing against young people in informal settlements, and the majority of those killed in the first year of the pandemic fit this demographic. But even aside from the killings, a number of people from these neighbourhoods were unjustly detained and fined, as the police took the mask mandate as an opportunity to expand their reign of terror.

The debate around masks is just one of the many ways the COVID-19 pandemic is forcing everyone to go back to the fundamentals of politics and society. We learn in "Introduction to Politics" classes about Enlightenment philosopher John Locke and the state of nature versus the state of man, and about French thinker Jean-Jacques Rousseau's social contract: citizens cede some of their personal freedoms to the state so that the state can be better positioned to protect the public good. The simple idea at the centre of living in a society—versus alone in a cabin in the forest at the mercy of animals, nature and other people—is that for some major issues, we are better off together than we are apart. Social life is a constant balancing act between personal freedoms and public obligations, which must constantly be adjusted in light of new information and developments.

So, if anything, the state of this debate is a strong indicator of the failures of basic civic education. What are societies for? What is government for? Both citizens and governments around the world seem to have lost sight of the basics and now are stuck in meaningless, cyclical debates around fundamentally irrational behaviour. It does not serve the public interest for citizens to use their personal freedom to jeopardise their own and other people's safety. But it similarly serves no one's interests for the government to use violence to inflict irreparable harm on citizens in the name of public health. Let's get back to a sober debate about working together to navigate this unprecedented time in global history.

5

WAITING TO BE SAVED

As COVID-19 raced its way across Africa in spring 2020, two stories were happening at once. The first was a story of governments using their armies and militarised police to beat, threaten and shoot their way to public health. This was the story of the Kenyan police killing more people than the disease in the week after the first recorded coronavirus case, and of a pregnant woman dying on the street because the Ugandan police would not let her motorcycle taxi take her to a hospital after curfew. It is the story of governments closing their borders too late, diverting money to security instead of hospitals, and waiting for someone from somewhere else to save them.

The second was a story of communities knitting together their meagre resources to fill the gap of failed services and absent states. It was the story of tailors across informal settlements in Nairobi and Mombasa sewing face masks out of scrap fabric and handing them out for free after price gouging by commercial suppliers. It was a young man renting speakers, tying them to his motorcycle, and riding through his neighbourhood to let people know about the new disease. It was translators offering their services without charge to put together public awareness campaigns in Somali, Maa, Zulu, Lingala, Fan Oromo or any of the thousands of other languages spoken across the continent. It was markets and small businesses making water jerricans available for mandatory hand-washing long before governments required it.

Almost as soon as the pandemic landed in Kenya, I was added to a Google group where young people from various parts of Kenya were volunteering to translate the WHO's messaging on the virus into local Kenyan languages, of which there are forty-four. We had all at this point received little bits of misinformation on social media, and I think the people who ran these groups sensed that if we waited for the government to rise to the challenge, the misinformation would have already taken root. The first case of COVID-19 in Kenya was confirmed on 13 March 2020. By April that year, accurate and timely public health messaging in many of Kenya's indigenous languages was not only available, but was being regularly broadcasted across the country.[1]

In August 2021, I rode my motorcycle over 800 kilometres across Kenya to the northernmost corner of Marsabit county. It was a personal catharsis to shake off the pandemic ennui that had settled on my shoulders, knowing that the motorcycle would force some of the social-distancing that the pandemic demanded, but that I would still have the benefit of proper ventilation because in the desert, no one really sleeps inside. On the first day of the ride back to Nairobi, I stopped at a small town called Moite—really no more than a cluster of thatched traditional houses on the banks of Lake Turkana. The only stone building was the local dispensary, which did not have a doctor and only had one nurse who came by from nearby Loiyangalani once or twice a week. I did not have mobile signal and hardly anyone spoke Kiswahili, Kenya's second national language, let alone English.

What I did find in Moite, however, were posters on the doors of the three town kiosks explaining how important hand-washing and social-distancing were for preventing the spread of COVID-19. Despite being on the periphery of the periphery of the periphery, the public health messages that had so far failed to be properly translated even in major urban centres in far wealthier countries had made their way here, and people were listening. This is the kind of thing that doesn't get captured when people collapse into preconfigured stories about why Africa must fail at managing the pandemic. The curative health-care system that provides treatment for people after they fall sick may be well and truly broken. But the preventive healthcare system is incredibly robust, because very few people can afford the cost of getting ill. Holistic preventative medicine, made up in no small part of effective communications networks and campaigns, is strong in so many parts of Africa because it has to be, and fighting the stigma and misinformation about the HIV/AIDS pandemic and the Ebola outbreak only drove more resources towards this, so that when COVID-19 happened, we did not have to start from zero.

Both of these stories about the pandemic in Africa are true, but only the first one is entering the archives of how Africa navigated the pandemic. Journalism, in general, is attuned to picking up lapses; even the best-intentioned media, premised on demanding accountability, can be biased towards reporting failures rather than successes. When confronted with a new situation, the punditry and analysis is inclined to pay attention to what is likely to go wrong rather than what might go right. But if only the first story enters the archive, the creativity and agency of vast swathes of humanity will be lost, with major consequences beyond the pandemic.

An archival record doesn't pick up everything, usually just what garners the most attention or is considered the most important. An archive, much like museums and other institutions that lay claim to being custodians of history, reflects the interests and predilections of those in power. Museums outside Africa are filled with masks and pots from the continent, not necessarily because Africans themselves thought these items were interesting, but because colonising armies and governments thought they were. A colonial archive would likely contain exhaustive records about a white district commissioner, down to the colour of his socks, but not the black woman who worked in his home. It's not because the latter is uninteresting or even unavailable for documentation; it is because those in power set the tone and the context for what goes into the archive, and subsequently, the stories that history will tell.

This makes the work that journalists and writers have been doing to tell the story of COVID-19 even more important. When it comes to Africa, we who write about the continent, and especially *from* the continent, know how hard it is to achieve an accurate representation of the state of society on platforms that have in-built tropes on deck and ready to launch. Africa is spoken for and spoken about, but so rarely allowed to speak, and this enables only a handful of meta-narratives to survive. We get PR-like tales of singular figures triumphant against all odds—the white saviour who braves malaria to deliver unprecedented interventions—or we get stories about the flailing state teetering on the edge of collapse. The relative weakness of African media outlets means that the complexities and nuances of what is happening away from power are rarely described, let alone analysed. The advent of digital media has gone some way towards opening up room for other narratives. Al Jazeera English has carved a global niche for deepening reporting from places outside the centres of power, and Africa Is a Country publishes critical takes on key issues. But digital archives are notoriously transient and even the most visible websites can disappear with the flick of a switch.

The archival record of the impact of the 1918 flu in Africa is an excellent example of how people understand agency and creativity within communities with constrained political power. It's not just about telling an accurate story. It's about how silences affect what people imagine is possible. When the official record of a community's history tells them that their ancestors did nothing when faced with near certain death, they tend to believe it and act like it's true.

In 1918, a strain of influenza that would come to be known as the "Spanish Flu" ravaged the world. Infected people lost significant lung function as the virus paved the way for bacterial pneumonia. Fluid and detritus accumulated in their lungs, and within days their skin turned blue and they died. By some estimates, the outbreak infected 500 million people—about one third of the world's population at the time—and took between 20 and 50 million lives, making it the second-deadliest pandemic in recorded history after the Black Death in the fourteenth century. Extreme estimates suggest that around 3 per cent of the world's population died, and the knock-on effects included significant political changes around the world. Coming at the end of World War I, the 1918 flu outbreak made that second decade of the twentieth century one of the deadliest in history.

The East Africa Protectorate, the British colony that would become the independent nation of Kenya, was not spared. After fighting for various European forces in World War I, African soldiers came home, bringing the disease into the territory. Many travelled inward along the Lunatic Express—the railway line that provided a route to the sea from Uganda, one of Britain's most profitable colonies of the time. A 2019 article estimated that on the Kenyan coast—the most urbanised and settled region of the fledgling country—the Spanish Flu killed 25.3 of every 1,000 people, less than the international average, but one of the deadliest recorded outbreaks in the territory.

Accurate information about the 1918 flu is difficult enough to come by in most countries, but in colonies like Kenya, the archival record is especially complicated. Much of what exists is from the perspective of colonial officers constructing a racist political state. So, the archives talk about how black people resisted many of the efforts at quarantine, portraying them as irrational, when in fact barring movement was one way the British created pools of forced labour.

In 1897, Queen Victoria declared the protectorate part of the British Empire, but until 1920, many ethnic groups fought back against the violence of colonisation with highly organised military campaigns. Between 1893 and 1911, the colonial administration was forced to launch twenty-eight major military operations in the territory, often aimed at suppressing communities that refused to collaborate with the colonisers. The official narrative on colonisation in Kenya tends to gloss over the depth and breadth of African resistance to the colonial project, but the fact is that much of the African population did not accept or even tolerate British imperialism.

Yet by 1915, the frequency of these operations had reduced, and the colonial government had begun putting in place the racist legislative structure for domination. Ethnic cantonment was the cornerstone of colonial oppression in Kenya, and severe punishments for leaving designated ethnic areas were a crucial part of turning free black men and women into prison labour. The Native Passes Regulation of 1900 and the Native Passes Ordinance of 1903 required Africans to have a pass to leave their own district. The 1906 Master and Servant Ordinance contained criminal penalties for black Africans in urban areas who left their work posts without authorisation.

In fact, six vagrancy ordinances were passed between 1898 and 1930, each designed to punish black people for their freedom of movement—and none applied to the white or Asian populations.

In 1915, the Native Registration Ordinance set in motion the *kipande* system, involving cruel and inhumane punishment for black men over the age of fifteen who did not carry a cumbersome document with their biometric details.

Why did the frequency and intensity of political resistance suddenly wane? On the one hand, Africans were dealing with unprecedented violence from the colonial administration. But they were also tackling outbreaks of diseases that had never been seen in the region before. European colonisers brought with them rinderpest, commonly known as cattle plague, which destroyed much of the indigenous cattle population, and jiggers, a small flea-like pest that burrows into feet, crippling the infected person and sometimes leading to gangrene. Bruce Berman and John Lonsdale, two historians specialising in Kenya's colonial era, estimate that the Maasai community, one of the most militant groups resisting the British in East Africa, may have lost up to 40 per cent of its population due to these two diseases.[2] Some historians argue that British colonial soldiers were only able to triumph over the Nandi resistance in the 1910s in Kenya because of the trypanosomiasis or sleeping sickness outbreak that eviscerated the community at around the same time. The pandemics and outbreaks in that first decade of the twentieth century decimated populations and made it impossible to mount any coordinated military resistance.

This is the context in which the quarantines and public health interventions to deal with the 1918 flu were deployed, but the archival record doesn't reflect this. Instead, it describes ignorant Africans disregarding the interventions of noble Europeans. Resistance to quarantine and enforced cantonment is framed as a rejection of public health initiatives, not as part of a broader campaign against the restrictions on freedom of movement placed on the African population. It certainly doesn't acknowledge a process in which scared and confused urban populations naturally sought the comfort of their extended families back in their ethnic cantons rather than face the full violence of the racist colonial state in the cities. The official story of how Africans behaved during the pandemic lacks empathy and nuance because those in power did not see Africans with empathy and nuance.

The archival record of Africa's experience with the 1918 flu is incomplete, because it is written by the colonisers who sought to present themselves as a benign force in an otherwise chaotic territory. Colonisation was a racist and violent enterprise couched in the language of a "civilising mission", and colonial archives of public health interventions—particularly those affecting freedom of movement—must be read against that reality.

The consequences of these partial archives still reverberate anywhere governments are drawing lessons from colonial public health practices. The pandemic violence in countries like India, Kenya, South Africa, Uganda and other settler colonies echoes the violence of the colonial state, in part because the successor independence governments saw the aggressive colonial interventions as logical and necessary. The archive presents violent policing responses as a natural part of a public health crisis response, and the successor governments don't question that.

The archive does not record the brutality of the *kipande* system that humiliated and properly assaulted Kenya's black population as a factor in why Africans may have resisted quarantine measures. As a result, the modern state may not realise that using police to enforce quarantine in informal settlements with a long history of police aggression may be opposed. The archive registers the problem not as a violent state clamping down on a society that they had been brutalising, but as the irrational resistance of "natives" against the well-meaning efforts of a righteous colonial state. The illusion that some violence is necessary to achieve public health goals because the "native" is inherently resistant to logic is passed down from colonisers and sustained because the archive is rarely critically interrogated.

Archives are not neutral; they're sites for contestation and projections of power. This is why historians from the Global South, like Brenda Sanya, a Kenyan feminist scholar, argue that questioning a nation's history as represented by the archive is absolutely necessary. An archive is a living thing in which what is explicit and what is silent are equally important. And critically for today, these records are silent on what Kenya's African population did to save themselves during the 1918 flu. Certainly, the traditional medical interventions that had been refined over centuries of community health practice must have struggled to respond to a novel virus.

But faced with widespread death and devastation, I don't believe that African communities did nothing other than wait for their oppressor to tap into their benevolent side. African traditional medicine had well-established practices for dealing with outbreaks of familiar diseases. For example, variolation, a precursor to modern-day vaccination in which healthy people were exposed to the blood of infected people to develop resistance to it, was recorded in Kenya, South Sudan, Nigeria and other parts of the continent. Community health structures existed and were often strong, but the colonising forces had no interest in them, as they were keen to promote the idea of superior European health systems.

The risk of diminishing the agency of African communities in this way persists. The HIV/AIDS pandemic has killed an estimated 40 million people globally, and Africa is one of the worst-affected regions. In Western Kenya, for example, the practice of wife inheritance, which leaders in some communities argue provided a social safety net for widows and orphans, created specific vulnerabilities where women whose partners died of HIV/AIDS transmitted the disease to their new partners and their families. In Kenya, HIV/AIDS hit communities that practiced wife inheritance through the 1990s hard. As long as African communities didn't understand the risk of HIV/AIDS, behaviour didn't change and the virus trounced societies. But communities learned, conduct changed and Western Kenyans now have robust non-medical responses to HIV/AIDS.

The same can be said of the Ebola outbreak of 2014. Projections that the epidemic would devastate the populations of the Mano River basin—Liberia, Sierra Leone, Guinea and Guinea Bissau—were confounded, not because a vaccine was developed or because the historically underfunded and ignored health systems magically transformed overnight. Community behaviour shifted the trajectory of the outbreak. People developed vocabularies for communicating the threat and the response to it, and funding and other forms of support went to frontline health workers who guided communities through the threat. Faced with novel and complex diseases, African communities did not sit back and wait for the disaster to destroy them. They rallied the best they could with whatever was available.

Which brings us back to the original challenge: what will the archives say that Africans did during the COVID-19 pandemic? Will the archives tell of foreigners coming in to help people who were already helping themselves? Or will the story of a wave of saviours from abroad frame Africans as passive recipients of external aid? How can we capture the complexity and agency of African communities in the face of this pandemic, without pandering to simplistic developmental narratives or diminishing the threat COVID-19 poses?

This is the task for writers covering Africa and the coronavirus: to hold space for the communities that those in power would rather not hear. It is a tremendous challenge. Very few African countries have media markets that can pay for quality independent investigative and documentary journalism. Many are dependent on Western donor governments to sustain their public health coverage, and this tips the scales in favour of stories that make those organisations look good. Other outlets operate as PR vehicles for their home governments and, by extension, for the countries that are their strong allies. Few foreign outlets are interested in true partnership with African journalists, and for the few critical journalists who exist, the erosion of press freedom across the continent is devouring whatever space they had to work.

But the archives of the twentieth-century pandemics, including HIV/AIDS, underscore how important it is for the first draft of history to rise to the challenge. Flawed and partial accounts of pandemics that understate the agency of affected communities and overstate the contribution of foreign interventions can have consequences long after the emergency period passes. People who don't see their agency and creativity valued in the official history of how they survived may give that agency away—making room for new eras of colonisation.

6

AIRBORNE

The pandemic made many of us start thinking about air in ways that we probably hadn't before—but maybe should have been. It made us think about the possibility that something so fundamental to our existence could turn out to be our weakest link, not because of the thing itself, but because of the way we had organised our lives around it. It made us realise how much time we spent inhaling recycled air (albeit at the perfect temperature) in closed spaces. If you live in a wealthy country, much of the air you breathe is recycled. You leave your air-conditioned house and walk to your air-conditioned bus or tram, or drive in your air-conditioned car, before arriving at your air-conditioned office, where you will spend the next eight to ten hours breathing recycled air.

A major reason why COVID-19 spread so fast in wealthy countries was because there was poor ventilation. Air conditioning is still relatively rare in Nairobi, but not as rare as it was ten years ago. The only air-conditioned spaces I enter in Nairobi on a normal week are the bank and perhaps a shopping mall, although most of my shopping will be done at an open-air market. But there are shopping malls cropping up on every street corner, designed to European specifications, with no windows that open and highly controlled air. Most new malls around the world follow a formula, and one piece of that formula is that fewer outside-facing windows mean that the people strolling around inside don't realise how much time they've spent there.

In Africa, the idea that fresh air is an asset is embedded in the most dramatic examples of African modernism. The best-designed buildings in Nairobi are constructed to breathe freely: the high ceilings that draw the air upwards in the City Market and the Kenyatta International Convention Centre, or the open slats on the side of the Kenya Coffee Producers and Traders Union building in the city's downtown. It is one of the unstated principles of the architectural style that air must be able to flow throughout the building, and that cooling and heating must not come from mechanical means.

This only works, of course, if the temperature outside the building remains pleasant. Unfortunately, the world is getting warmer, and more of us are reaching for air conditioning as a solution to the problem; just over 110 million air-conditioning units were sold in 2019, the year before the pandemic hit.[1] Never mind the fact that the use of air conditioners running on electricity generated by fossil fuels is a significant contributor to climate change. Access to controlled air is still viewed a major indicator of how developed a country is. It is implied that the ability to tame the weather and keep it outside, and to subjugate it to our whims, is the measure of how much progress we have made as a society. Pity those poor souls whose lives are still subject to the vagaries of the weather.

I kept this in mind as I watched the debate about ventilation unfold in the West, particularly in schools, where policymakers started to notice that children spend an inordinate amount of time not breathing fresh air. The idea of controlling the air as a marker of progress got turned on its head when the air itself became the main way through which the disease was transmitted. In the USA, one representative of the Environmental Protection Agency (EPA) called COVID-19 a sort of "hallelujah moment" because she had been fighting for years to get the government to notice that so many schools in the country had terrible air quality and children were getting asthma from mould, or sharing colds and flus at an incredible rate.[2] Once scientists figured out that controlled air was part of the problem, there was a great push in many countries to retrofit classrooms with air filters so that children could get back to class.

It is a bad thing that so many African children still study outside. We should be investing more in education and building the kind of schools that celebrate the love that we have for our children. Children should be able to learn in pleasant environments. It is a bad thing that education is not the most important thing that so many of African governments spend money on.

But perhaps one reason why African children have largely been spared the worst of the pandemic is that so many of them do not regularly breathe controlled air. The weather allows for it. The windows remain open across many countries of the continent unless there's a rainstorm. Certainly, in Kenya, the average Kenyan simply does not spend that much time indoors. Farmers and herders will only return home to sleep and, in some communities, only after several days out to pasture. There are buildings where the fight between man and mosquito, or the choice between stale air and malaria, has led people to seal up vents, but for the most part, even those of us who work indoors rarely breathe controlled air.

The EPA, by contrast, found that Americans spend an average of 90 per cent of their time inside;[3] a 2013 study by the WHO reported the same results for people in Europe.[4] I can't find the data on African countries, not even specific countries.

STRANGE AND DIFFICULT TIMES

All I have is story. African countries like South Africa and Egypt that were worst hit by the pandemic are united by the fact that they both experience extreme weather conditions, and controlled air is more common. In Egypt, air conditioning helps people manage extreme heat; in South Africa, there is extreme cold, and so people are more likely to spend their time indoors. But while extreme heat is certainly increasingly common across the continent, most of us are still dependent on finding ways to exist in harmony with the open air, rather than trying to battle it directly. Hotels, banks, malls and airports rely on controlled air, but the majority of us are not spending extended periods of time in those places. If this is indeed a major factor in the spread of the disease, why is it then easier for people to believe that the low rate of transmission across the continent is somehow miraculous?

It is this unseeing that drives me in part to start to pay more attention to the rhymes and rhythms of the pandemic than I probably should. I am not a scientist. This is not my core work. I am a person who watches people and events and tries to see the things that the mainstream media would rather not see. It is interesting to me that when talking about why the worst of the pandemic has, at the time of writing, skipped the continent, there is a rush towards one of two answers: that Africans are either innately miraculous beings or that we are lying about the extent to which the disease has affected the continent (see Chapter 10). Neither of these theories have sufficient explanatory power.

This idea that Africans are inherently magical creatures bothers me deeply. In his essay "Concerning Violence," Frantz Fanon writes something about the relationship between superstition and responses to colonial violence that I find deeply compelling here:

> In [colonised countries,] the occult sphere is a sphere belonging to the community which is entirely under magical jurisdiction. ... Believe me, the zombies are more terrifying than the settlers; and in

consequence the problem is no longer that of keeping oneself right with the colonial world and its barbed-wire entanglements, but of considering three times before urinating, spitting, or going out into the night.

The supernatural, magical powers reveal themselves as essentially personal; the settler's powers are infinitely shrunken, stamped with their alien origin. We no longer really need to fight against them [the colonists] since what counts is the frightening enemy created by myths. We perceive that all is settled by a permanent confrontation on the phantasmic plane.[5]

There is an intangible something that makes it necessary to invoke magic and exception instead of finding practical reasons for why Africa is having a different experience of the pandemic. Fanon thought that it allowed the colonised person to rise above the constant violence of colonisation, to fight a battle that can be won—against the supernatural enemy of myth, rather than the colonial brutality of reality. During the pandemic, we as Africans experienced all kinds of systemic violence: we were summarily excluded by unjust global travel bans, we were denied access to medicines that were freely available elsewhere, and we were abandoned by leaders who would not speak up for us when we urgently needed them to. And so, we are perhaps too quick to grasp hold of the idea that if we are somehow managing to stay afloat during this time of intense crisis, it must be on a plane in which the odds are not so clearly stacked against us.

Fanon's ideas help me rationalise things, even if it still bothers me that so many people (including some within the continent) think that if Africans are succeeding at something that is devastating other people, it must be a result of something ineffable, rather than a product of our actions. It's part of a broader dehumanising narrative that creates an excuse for people not to help when help is needed. It provides justification for the idea that sending vaccines to Africa is simply not a priority, because we will never be as badly affected. I'm not a scientist so I cannot offer a scientific explanation of what is happening, but I get stuck on this point: why is it easier to believe that Africans are inherently magical, or that we are lying about the scale of our deaths, than to look into the fact that our lives are simply different? Not worse or better, but simply different.

The air quality question stayed with me, because one year into the pandemic, I had to start travelling again. It was March 2021, and vaccines were not yet widely available on the continent, so I had to develop a risk management strategy. Because of the political choices made very early on by the governments of the most powerful countries in the world—to lie about the nature of the disease, to refuse to make the hard choices needed to slow its spread—the pandemic was not going away as promised. The "before" was gone, but the "after" was not yet guaranteed, so it became necessary to find a way to live with the virus at that time. For me, this meant getting back to travel, and I needed a plan.

I found myself thinking more and more about the air that I was breathing, and how to mitigate the risks it posed. The plan was simple: keep your mask on in places where there are crowds and where there is controlled air; take your mask off in the fresh air and where people are not densely packed together. And this is when I began to notice that in Kenya, I am more likely to be in places where it's okay to lower the mask—walking to the market, eating at outdoor restaurants, etc. Public transport is a risk, but even then, the windows would be wide open and we weren't breathing controlled air. But when overseas, I was breathing recycled air on the train, on the plane, in the subway, in the hotel, in the conference centre ... The only brief moments of fresh air were the walks from the airport doors to the bus stop.

Most of Africa continues to see low rates of extreme illness from COVID-19, even though there is a suggestion that the actual figures may be higher than announced. Where is the comparative science on the amount of time that people of different professions or social communities spend indoors or outdoors? All I have right now is story—I want to see proof. This is the kind of study that an African research institute could do which could actually affect how the world understands the pandemic and what we do in response to it. It could be a low-cost way for African scientists to make their mark on global science. But I have no power to suggest this to anyone; all I can do is write and tweet about it in the hope that a scientist somewhere sees it as worthwhile. And now I am stuck in another loop of thought about the state of science on the continent: the tyranny of certain ontologies and epistemologies that lead so many brilliant people to think that research can only be one thing. That our contributions to knowledge will only matter if we can also develop our own vaccines and build our own highly expensive genomics labs. That science and knowledge have to be large, expensive and elaborate in order to matter. But the context in which disease happens and is understood is also research and is also science. Learning how what we have contributes to how things are going is also science.

Dependent on funding from overseas research councils and waiting to be brought in as secondary investigators on foreign research projects, our scientists are stuck answering other people's questions first instead of answering our own. Granted, at the beginning of the pandemic, there was a lot of ambiguity about the role of ventilation in the control of COVID-19. I myself was convinced by the WHO's initial statements that the coronavirus was not transmitted by air particles but by droplets, and so, in that regard, masks made little sense. Once it became apparent that the disease was in fact airborne, it was strange to me that we still couldn't get this comparative data on how much time people were spending outdoors and why this mattered.

And so, we got stuck in this hygiene theatre, having to practically wipe ourselves down with sanitiser before entering air-conditioned malls and banks. We had our temperatures checked, even though eventually this turned out to be a waste of time and technology. When a simpler and cheaper thing we could have been doing was opening the windows and making it easier for people to spend more time outdoors. There is an embedded logic in there about hierarchies of knowledge to which we must pay attention. When things go wrong at the scale that they have with this pandemic, there is often an instinct to reach for the most complicated solution, but sometimes the simplest ones can illuminate a pathway out so much better. And we didn't just reach for the more complicated solutions: we as Africans routinely berated ourselves for not being able to answer questions based on conditions experienced elsewhere, instead of surveying the terrain and asking the simpler questions which were arising organically from our own contexts. We wanted, and many still want, a genetic answer for why the disease was sparing us. We wanted expensive science that would put us in the foreign streams of knowledge, instead of practical knowledge that would help us live in the new reality the disease created.

And so, we will continue to build malls, banks, airports and the like which depend on recycled air, because the prevailing belief is that breathing controlled air equals progress, even while other countries' experiences with recycled air—its environmental costs and its connection to respiratory disease—suggest that a different way might be better. We continue to reject styles of architecture designed to let more air in, in favour of glass towers that act as greenhouses and need controlled air to remain usable. We keep thinking about the air in ways that are not consistent with the way the air behaves, trying to bottle the wind.

7

GLOBAL

We are also the world.

I think I should get it tattooed somewhere on my body, or printed on my business cards, because I have to say it so often. We are also the world. Even today, the phrase "the world" is deployed with such alarming consistency to mean "rich countries" or "Western countries" and not the nearly 8 billion of us who share this planet. And so, we "vaccinated the world", even though most of Africa remains unvaccinated. "The world" has been moving on from COVID-19 in 2022, even while millions of people across the planet are still picking up the pieces after the havoc wreaked by the disease. "The world" is used as a convenient shorthand to mean "the people that we think matter", and not simply "the people".

We find ourselves listening more to the people who have the most power instead of listening to each other properly, regardless of where we are in the global hierarchy. We hear a narrative about "the world" as imagined by those who have the most power within it and we accept it as truth, even when that version of the story does us an injustice. This means that even when other people are getting the wrong end of the stick when it comes to understanding how our lives are organised, we begin by embracing their perspectives on who we are and what we contribute, instead of looking at ourselves fairly. It means that when the international news tells us that "the world" is reeling from something or moving on from something, we accept that, even though if we looked across at our neighbourhoods, our communities or the countries next door, we might see things a little differently. It also means that, too often, we in Africa are primed to believe the worst version of ourselves and the best version of other people; when something bad happens, we are quicker to blame ourselves than the systems in which we exist.

During the pandemic, many Africans were quick to accept a version of the story that said that their countries were inherently given to failure and that whatever disaster came to pass, we had somehow invited it. This is qualitatively different from necessary criticism about corruption, misallocated funds or governments that spend more on the presidential travel budget than they do on public health. Because looking across the various oceans, we could easily see that these were not uniquely African problems. They were challenges that all types of countries faced. The UK was involved in a corruption scandal over misallocated personal protective equipment contracts (see Chapter 19). And a US think tank pointed out that under the Trump administration, at least twenty-seven companies connected to the president received up to US $10.5 billion in lobbying funds from the government during the pandemic, including companies associated with the president's son-in-law.[1]

This doesn't negate the fact that corruption in the COVID-19 response globally was a problem. If anything, it restates that it was an international problem. But it does negate the idea that this is an "African" problem that justifies denying Africans access to lifesaving medicines. It rejects a harmful exceptionalism that can only understand Africa through the lens of pity.

When the fight to vaccinate the world began, I found myself routinely in conversations with people generally, and with Africans particularly (both online or in person), who were convinced that the reason vaccines were not being distributed to African countries was because our governments were uniquely terrible and that we had brought the misfortune on ourselves. We had brought it on ourselves because we failed to vote properly, ignoring the systems that force bad governments upon us. We deserved to suffer because we refused to rise up against these governments, ignoring the fact that the Sudanese people have been revolting continuously for more three years and have received nothing for their protest but killings, arrests and the condescending detachment of "the world".

It's worth stating that this is different from a desire to hold African governments accountable where they do fail. No one is more critical of African governments when they fail than I am, and accountability is a crucial response to a collective disaster like the pandemic. I keep coming back to Frantz Fanon because he has said so many things that hold true for this moment. In *The Wretched of the Earth*, he insists that the "heads of the government are the true traitors in Africa, for they sell their country to the most terrifying of all its enemies: stupidity".[2] We know that we have terrible leadership. But we are also the world, and this does not explain all the disparate outcomes, nor justify the idea that our suffering is acceptable. And if people in other parts of the world should not be singled out for suffering because of the quality of their leadership, why should Africans be treated any differently? The search is not for magical absolution that says that African governments must not be held accountable for the losses they create. The search is for a fair perspective on what it means to be part of "the world"—what flaws and shortcomings exist across all the different forms of social organisation.

It is strange to me that the Global South is routinely overlooked in the description of what "the world" is doing in response to anything. Even well-meaning people, when trying to raise awareness of a crisis or a situation that dominates their local media, will routinely ask "why isn't the world saying anything about this?" even if African countries have been vocal about it. The geopolitical anxieties of China and the United States are routinely framed as desires to see "the world" behave in certain ways, even though most of the world will not benefit, except in the most abstract way, no matter who wins that particular battle of wills. This means that even those places which are not contemplated within this idea of "the world" routinely see themselves not in relation to their own communities but as extensions of that mythical "world". This must be why so many Kenyans got caught up in the geopolitical debates about whether we should accept Chinese vaccines or Western vaccines, more invested in the power battle between these two enemies than in our own survival. We don't like to think of ourselves as among the ones who are being excluded from the story about "the world".

This pandemic should have taught us all that, by the logic of this system, all Africans are equally expendable. We are not among the number when "the world" is choosing who is going to survive. We like to believe that we are also the world, but this pandemic has reminded us that we are not automatically counted in it. It sounds particularly grim, but it really isn't. It's a moment of earnest and honest reflection that should fuel a different perspective on how we do politics and how we respond to a changing world. It should be liberating to discover that we have agency over the course of our futures. We don't have to tether our survival to the benevolence of "the world"; we are also the world, and we can choose to survive on our own terms.

African countries spent the better part of 2021 begging for medicine and being told in no unsubtle terms that the survival of the West specifically, but wealthier countries in general, was more important than working together to survive the pandemic.

African governments raised the money to pay for medicine but were undercut by wealthier countries buying obscenely more than they needed, only to end up throwing much of it away. England, which purchased up to three times the number of vaccines it needed (even while refusing to share doses with poor countries), had thrown away 4 per cent of all the doses it had, or 4.7 million, by October 2021.[3] Canada had discarded at least 1 million doses by the end of 2021, at a time when around 47 per cent of the world's population had yet to receive a single dose.[4]

"Vaccinate the world" turned out to mean "Vaccinate 'the world'".

But this narrow version of the story overlooks the fact that for the first time in recent history, African countries looked around and realised that all we had was each other. We are losing the part of the story where Africa delivered a masterclass in regional organisation because "the world" simply was not coming.

On 17 March 2021, during a hearing updating the US House Foreign Affairs Committee on Africa's preparedness for the COVID-19 pandemic, Dr John N. Nkengasong, current head of the Africa Centres for Disease Control and Prevention (Africa CDC), which coordinates the political and medical responses to disease outbreaks across the continent, dropped an interesting fact that remains woefully underreported.[5] "In February 2020," he said, "no African country had the capacity to test for COVID-19. By the end of March [that year], every single country on the continent had the capacity to test for COVID-19. That is remarkable". While "the world" was preparing for a tragedy in Africa, Africans were on the move. The simplest explanation was the governments decided to step aside and let the experts lead the way, and the result was a remarkable triumph for regional coordination on the continent.

Regional coordination isn't a thing that most of us think about on an ordinary basis. Most of the time, multinational organisations are discussed in a negative light—for all the ways they fail to intervene when they are needed most and the many ways they strain already distressed budgets. But when an international disaster like a pandemic happens, regional coordination becomes a crucial step in breaking down the paths of action into conceivable or attainable measures.

So, it mattered that in the worst moments of the pandemic, Africa did something that almost no other region of the world managed to accomplish: it worked together. In the same week that the African Union was making submissions to the US House Foreign Affairs Committee, the European Union was considering suspending exports of vaccines made in Europe because its own vaccination effort had been significantly disrupted by alleged hoarding from the US and the UK.[6] Indeed, EU member state Hungary opted out of the Union's procurement deal with Pfizer and BioNTech, instead using vaccines from Russia and China, in addition to other Western jabs.[7]

Meanwhile, throughout 2021, the United States continued to hoard an obscene excess of vaccines even while neighbouring countries in the Americas, including Canada, struggled to secure delivery of doses they had paid for.[8] The Association of Southeast Asian Nations was perhaps the only other region in the world that demonstrated a heightened level of coordination in response to the pandemic.[9] Even within international bodies like the WHO, COVID-19 has been a significant test for the idea of working multilaterally.

The success of regional coordination in Africa doesn't fit simplistic narratives of why the continent is muddling through despite the expectation of failure. Not that the responses have been perfect, or that there have not been grave losses, but the failure that "the world" was waiting on has not yet materialised. And a big reason why the African COVID-19 response has been so remarkable is that it has to be, because when disaster strikes, "the world" does not always respond with solidarity.

When Ebola broke out in West Africa in 2014, many of the outcomes that people feared did in fact take place. The public healthcare systems of the worst-affected country buckled and all but collapsed in the face of the novel disease. Initially, there was no regional approach to the problem—only ad hoc acts of support and solidarity from various governments and international organisations like Médecins Sans Frontières. There was anxiety around the novel disease and people lied about being infectious. Secret burials were conducted to avoid stigma. People avoided going to hospital because they thought that it was making their loved ones ill.[10] Borders were shut against the countries where the disease was most prevalent, but in some cases against the entire continent, which was believed to be contagious by affiliation.[11]

During the COVID-19 pandemic, only one of these factors remained unchanged. Realising in the wake of the Ebola epidemic that regional coordination was a huge blind spot, in 2017, the African Union, alongside other partners, officially launched the Africa CDC. The Africa CDC provides timely support to national public health institutions to help them respond quickly to disease threats. In addition to policy work, it runs free webinars and briefings for scientists and journalists which are also open to the public and streamed on every available platform. The lesson of the 2014 Ebola outbreak was clear: there is significant human capital in Africa that can make a huge difference if institutions invest it where it is needed.

As someone who is not a health expert, but who was deeply concerned about how we collectively survive this new disease, being able to tune into these briefings from the comfort of my own home and on my social media account was a lifeline. Some people like to run into burning buildings without understanding why the building is on fire; I like knowing what caused the fire even if I'm not sure how I will survive it. The briefings from the Africa CDC were not as well attended as press conferences by presidents and political leaders. But they taught me more about COVID-19 and the pandemic as a systemic challenge than many other sources of information. More importantly, they were a lesson in what Africans could build together if we let the experts do what they needed to do with the support they required.

There are two other pieces of the regional response that risk getting lost in the official story of what Africa did when COVID-19 hit. The Africa Vaccine Acquisition Task Team was a group headed up by various Africans with a high profile on the continent—entrepreneurs, economists and other public figures—to figure out how to buy vaccines for the continent after the international system failed.[12] It is a branch of the Africa CDC that responds directly to the needs set before it by its parent body. It might get lost in history that African countries needed these platforms because COVAX, the multilateral system, failed spectacularly.

COVAX is an initiative of the Global Vaccine Alliance (Gavi), which is a public–private partnership supporting research into and distribution of vaccines against seventeen infectious diseases. Gavi in turn is a partnership between private philanthropy like the Bill and Melissa Gates Foundation and vaccine manufacturers, as well as multilateral organisations like UNICEF and the World Health Organization. The logic of COVAX was actually pretty straightforward: if all countries pitched in and bought vaccines according to their needs and capacities, as well as with some philanthropic support, the organisation could not only provide the funding needed to accelerate vaccine development, but it could also get jabs to the people who needed them most.[13] It sounds simple enough, but it only works if the vision of "the world" is shared by everyone who participates, and it became clear early on that this was not the case.

Wealthy countries gobbled up the global distribution of vaccines on two fronts. First, they entered into agreements with the various vaccine manufacturers to purchase doses even before they left the conveyor belt.[14] At a 2021 Africa CDC briefing, I heard the CEO of vaccine manufacturer Moderna tell attendees that he had no extra vaccines in any of his factories; as soon as doses were made, they were packaged up and loaded onto trucks for distribution to rich nations. But these countries then also flexed their economic muscles to acquire vaccines from within the COVAX system itself, instead of leaving them for the countries for which bilateral deals with vaccine producers were simply not feasible. Médecins Sans Frontières argues that Gavi simply gave the private companies too much power to shape how the manufacture and distribution of jabs would go,[15] and they designed it to maximise profit.

One thing that certainly didn't change between the Ebola epidemic and the COVID-19 outbreak was the speed with which "the world" moved to shut Africa out. In the early days of the pandemic, I, too, was reluctant to urge border closures, in part because I did not want to articulate a politic that reinforced the borders defining so much of the systemic violence inflicted against Africans. Particularly against Chinese people, the arguments for shutting frontiers were often laced with racist undertones. However, as border closures grew more common, it became clear that very few countries were willing to ban travel by Europeans, even when COVID-19 was at its worse in this continent. Kenya officially closed its borders to international travel in May 2020 but reopened them in August that year. In January 2021, Kenya waived the mandatory quarantine for travellers from the UK, even though the UK kept its own mandatory quarantine for so-called "red-list countries" (which by the end were only African countries) until December 2021.[16]

African countries and African people had learnt from the Ebola pandemic and had developed mechanisms to protect their populations from new diseases. But "the world" had learnt nothing about African people.

None of this changes the fact that African countries still need to do more to build up their healthcare systems. None of this changes the fact that even this regionally coordinated response could have been improved if it had met strong healthcare systems. But two things can be true at the same time, and holding on to that complexity is crucial to make sure that the story is told properly. The idea that poor people generally, but African people specifically, would do nothing to defend themselves against grave illness is a deeply racist one. It's not just the belief that we can't; it's also the belief that we won't, as if we somehow value our existence less.

The pandemic has changed something in the way that African people see their position in "the world", and global politics has changed perhaps irreversibly as a result. But it's not just about how the vaccines were distributed. It's also about the way in which institutions that were supposed to function for the benefit everyone responded. Not enough people paid attention to the global economic conversation to realise that African countries were getting cheated. In September 2021, President Félix Tshisekedi of the Democratic Republic of Congo, in his capacity as the head of the African Union at that time, asked the International Monetary Fund (IMF) to issue Special Drawing Rights (SDRs), basically a tool to give money from a common pool of currencies to countries that are struggling economically.[17] SDRs are not issued regularly. They are a way of increasing liquidity or giving countries money to spend on important things, in recognition that something seriously wrong.[18]

The IMF could have issued SDRs to the countries that were struggling the most and asked wealthier countries to share with them, particularly given that many poor countries had been forced to allocate resources towards the pandemic response when the containment strategies of richer nations failed. Remember that the pandemic spread in part because the wealthy did not act swiftly enough to prevent it. So, it matters that the bulk of the SDRs issued in 2021 went to wealthier countries instead of poorer ones.[19] It deepened the feeling that the pandemic was going to function as a massive reallocation of resources from those who had little to those who already had more than they needed. The year 2022 also began with demands from these same organisations that poor countries in Africa, Asia and South America subject their economies to austerity measures in order to access the liquidity that the SDRs could have created. Kenyan economist David Ndii likes to say that "only Africa is subjected to economic orthodoxy". Perhaps not only Africa, but certainly only poor countries must submit their economies to textbook theories about how the world should respond to various issues, while richer nations continue to behave as if they are the exception to every rule.

Maybe the biggest difference between how the injustice played out this time around and how it has played out in the past is that now, thanks to digital media, they are not just well documented, but easily understood. It's not so much that the pandemic has changed the way world politics works; it's that for the first time in history, more of us are witness to it. More of us see the inequalities and more of us are unwilling to quietly accept them, even if it is not necessarily clear at this moment what "the world" will do in response to this great act of witnessing.

When people talk about "the world" in global politics, they are usually referring to how powerful countries relate to each other. But what makes countries powerful is the amount of power that smaller countries are willing to cede to them. It's about the space that smaller countries make for larger countries to project their power into their natural terrain. Witnessing this moment of intense failure has completely undermined the logic that making room for powerful nation, so that they in turn can extend their "protection" or "solidarity", is a good approach. The world—the *real* world, as in the global majority—is less likely to accept mainstream arguments about why certain things must happen the way they do, and that changes things. More and more countries want true fairness, even though right now there is no clear sense of what that fairness might look like; more and more people are calling out the failings of a global system that is founded on the idea that only a handful of countries must survive and the rest of us must just roll the dice and hope that luck runs in our favour.

The cruelty and arrogance that Western countries in particular, but also wealthier countries in general, have shown the rest of us in the way drugs were produced and distributed around the world has fundamentally shifted something that may never shift back. The scars from this moment in history have caused the kind of seismic geopolitical movement that can alter the course of history. It's already evident in the way African countries have been reluctant to engage directly with the war in Ukraine, much to the chagrin of European and American leaders, who seem alarmed by the idea that Africa may be unhitching its horses from the Western wagon. It's becoming clearer to more and more of the people of the global majority that when Western governments talk about "the world", they are not talking about us, and that is already altering calculations about how to respond to the changing global situation.

In international law we use the phrase "constitutive practices" to refer to a set of behaviours that collectively infuse meaning into a geographical entity or society. So, citizens participate in democracy, but participating in democracy is a constitutive practice that defines citizenship—it is the doing of democracy that gives meaning to the idea of being a citizen. In the end, what saved African countries from the worst of the pandemic was solidarity—looking around and realising that we had greater chances of survival together than in waiting for "the world" to act.

GLOBAL

Solidarity is a beautiful constitutive practice to give meaning to the idea of "Africa", and it stands in remarkable contrast to the way "the world" is used to stratify and divide people into sets of who matters, who matters less and who matters not at all. I am always wary of this label "Africa" because it is so regularly used as a shorthand or euphemism for "black", "poor" or simply "Other". In too many minds, the idea of "Africa" can only be processed through a lens of pity, and so I've always been reluctant to unreservedly embrace it. But maybe the pandemic will force "the world" to see things a little differently.

8

POLICING A PANDEMIC

Monday, 6 April 2020 marked the ten-day anniversary of Kenya's dawn-to-dusk lockdown. With at least six deaths connected to the curfew, the authorities had already killed as many if not more people than the virus, and police brutality remained an alarming constant until March 2022, when the last remaining restrictions were eased in the country.[1] On the first night of confinement, social media in Kenya was full of videos of police officers using teargas against ferry passengers, beating traders at marketplaces, harassing drivers and overall menacing the public in the name of maintaining order. When challenged, the then Cabinet Secretary for Health, Mutahi Kagwe, declined to condemn the violence outright, instead urging civilians to avoid "placing themselves in situations where they might be confronted by the police". Regardless of the nature of the threat and its significance, it seemed that the government of Kenya could only resort to the most unsophisticated tool in its arsenal—the violence of the police.

The policing of the pandemic was a brutal show of arrogance and force visited primarily on poor, male bodies, but really on anyone who could be killed. The youngest victim, thirteen-year-old Yassin Moyo, was standing on the balcony of his family home in the first week of the curfew, watching the police teargas poor people to get them to enter their houses before sunset, when he was shot in the stomach by a police officer.[2] He died on the way to hospital. In September 2021, brothers Benson Njiru Ndwiga and Emmanuel Marura Ndwiga, twenty-two and nineteen respectively, were on their way home from a butcher's shop they had just opened with their father when they were arrested by police for allegedly violating lockdown rules.[3] Their bodies were found in the morgue two days later.

One remarkable feature of the politics of the novel coronavirus was how starkly it seemed to exacerbate whatever structural inequalities it found in the societies it entered. In Kenya, police violence has been a regular feature of public life for years, particularly in informal settlements. According to the Independent Medico-Legal Unit, a non-profit which collects data on police brutality and supervises independent autopsies in suspected cases of police violence, the Kenyan authorities killed 189 people between October 2018 and September 2019.[4] The average age of those killed was twenty-eight, and in 75 per cent of those cases, the police alleged that the victims were criminals and thugs, even where there was compelling evidence to the contrary.

So, even from the beginning of the curfew, individuals in informal settlements were already on edge, not least because of the loss of income that the lockdown created. Residents were also concerned that public order measures would lead to even more arbitrary violence, particularly against a population that was facing the choice between death by illness and death by starvation. Like many other countries, Kenya gave the police force increased power to implement restrictions to tackle COVID-19. These rules, contained in the Public Order Act, gave officers unprecedented powers to detain, arrest and fine. But in addition to these formal systems, police were also filmed using corporal punishment and teargas without any perceptible threat, which is, of course, illegal.

Historically, public order restrictions have been applied where there was a threat to state security—such as during the attempted coup of August 1982—or where there is a threat of insurgency, as in the Mount Elgon region. (Active between 2005 and 2008, the Sabaot Land Defence Force militia group was ostensibly formed to resist efforts to evict squatters near the second-highest mountain in Kenya, although in the process they killed at least 600 civilians. In response, the government, under the cover of numerous public order laws, used the army against civilians and members of the group. Exact numbers of those detained, tortured and killed by soldiers remain unclear, but human rights groups put the estimates in the thousands.) But this was first time that such laws were invoked to manage a public health crisis. And the Kenyan government did not seem to have unpacked the qualitative difference between suppressing a rebellion and reducing the risk of an outbreak, because the pattern of behaviour was exactly the same.

Aside from the clear ethical issues of police officers abusing their power, the unprecedented police crackdown posed another risk: if extreme measures were applied without due caution and consideration, they would eventually be resisted. Experts warned that because so many countries had failed to act decisively in the early days of the coronavirus outbreak, lockdowns and curfews would likely be with us for a long time. Widespread rejection of containment measures could lead to wholesale social and economic collapse in countries that did not have the public health capacity to deal with a large outbreak of a highly infectious disease. We needed the public to comply and modify their behaviour, whether or not Big Brother was watching.

Globally, police brutality was a major secondary risk to the public created by COVID-19. Kenya is one example, but across the developing world—in India, Uganda, South Africa, Egypt and many other countries—states disintegrated into arbitrary violence against civilians under the guise of enforcing curfews and stay-at-home orders. But consent is crucial to fostering compliance with open-ended and strict physical-distancing measures. Much like with the racist policing of the past, violence may deliver short-term submission, but it will not be enough to maintain order once the public realises that they vastly outnumber the police. What will we do with the people if they don't understand why they must stay home?

What hope can possibly be salvaged from such a cruel narrative of an institution so seemingly committed to serving as an agent of death? Not much, overall. The tragedy of the Kenyan police is that of incomplete decolonisation: an institution built in 1920, primarily to protect the property and personhood of white settler families as they invaded the land and oppressed the black population that lived on it, did not change when the country became independent. Instead, it found new purpose in protecting the interests of the rich. It's the tragedy of institutions designed to exact violence on black people being taken over by black people and continuing to do the same. In "Concerning Violence", Frantz Fanon explains how police officers and the police station were the dividing line between the settler and the colonised: "the policeman and the soldier, by their immediate presence and their frequent and direct action[,] maintain contact with the native and advise him by means of rifle butts and napalm not to budge. ... [T]he agents of government speak the language of pure force."[5] The inherent purpose of the police to use force to impose the appearance of order on the oppressed doesn't change because the oppressor is black: the machine continues to tick on in the logic for which it was built. It sees poor black people as a threat because it is trained on and oriented around that fear.

The thin sliver of hope, if there is one in this context, is the sheer number of Kenyans who are finally attuned to this reality.

None of us are born abolitionists or questioners of institutions. As children, we are raised to accept certain truths about the world and not necessarily to be intentional or deliberate in thinking about why. Indeed, there are many adults who interpret their role in a child's life as getting them to stop asking "why?" So, it means something when a critical mass of adults starts to ask this question. When I first returned to Kenya in 2015 after spending some time working in Madagascar, I wrote a number of articles about police brutality, and was generally met with the response, "well, they are all criminals" or "they deserved what they got". As most of the victims of police violence come from slums and are away from the middle- and upper-class gaze, the crime narrative is rarely challenged. But the small sliver of hope that has come out of the pandemic is that growing numbers of people reject this narrative and are pushing back against it. A coalition of local Kenyan rights groups sued the police in September 2020 for their violence during the lockdown. People came out in large numbers to protest it, led by activists like Juliet Wanjira.[6] It is a small star in a dark night sky, but it still points to the possibility that we can do things differently.

Policing in many parts of the world was already broken, and much like with other urgent questions around governance priorities, COVID-19 provided an opportunity for countries to reflect on what the purpose of the institution is. The objective of the movement restrictions around the world was for people to modify their behaviour quickly, and to stop situations that heighten the risk of contracting COVID-19. The public is not the enemy here, the virus is, and we need informed consent to get the kind of wholesale compliance needed to tackle this pandemic and any future ones. Using the police as a substitute for effective public health communication and awareness not only makes this work more difficult; it undermines it completely.

9

THE FEARS OF THE GLOBAL MINORITY

Travellers from *those* countries are entering our countries.

Other countries are preventing our travellers from entering.

African borders are too open to control the flow of disease. (Coming from the region with the most open borders in the world.)

Borders are open elsewhere. (Our open borders are different.)

Asian people are wearing masks in public. (Minding their own business, but still Asian people.)

Children will be traumatised by making them wear masks in school. (But not that children will die.)

> *They* will be unable to use the vaccines properly.
> *They* will be unable to make vaccines.
> *They* will be unable to distribute vaccines safely.
> *They* will be unable to find fridges to store vaccines.
> *They* will be unable to pay.
> *They* don't know enough to do the work that needs doing.
> *They* will all end up here when things fall apart *there*.
> *They* will make *us* sick.
> *They* will bring the disease *here*.

DEATH

10

THE ART OF ASKING USEFUL QUESTIONS

"Why aren't more Africans dying of the coronavirus?"

Almost every major international news outlet has asked a variation of that question. Some speculated that something structural or physiological has dampened the impact of COVID-19 on Africa's population; otherwise, Africa would be faring worse. Others argued that African governments are simply doing a better job of managing the disease than other regions, despite ample evidence to the contrary. Neither reflects the complex realities of COVID-19 in Africa.

The question itself, in its crudest form, provoked considerable, justifiable anger on social media in various African countries. Yet as the deaths mounted in Brazil, India and the United States, and even as Europe prepared for its nth wave of contagion, the official per capita death toll in Africa has remained the lowest of all the continents. Just over 184 deaths per million had been recorded in Africa by the time of writing, compared to 310 in Asia, 384 in Oceania, and a staggering 2,488 in North America, 2,528 in Europe and 3,038 in South America. In total, just over a quarter of a million deaths have been reported in Africa's official figures, far lower than every other continent on the planet, bar the much less populous Oceania. Even in South Africa, the most severely affected African country, confirmed deaths are far fewer than predicted. Experts are indeed wondering why their forecasts were wrong. But wondering why forecasts were wrong is very different from asking a crude question outside of a research context. The more vulgar formulation relates to the ways that knowledge about Africa is constructed, and the loaded, false premises that lead to framing important issues in partial and violent ways. After all, to ask why more Africans aren't dying of COVID-19 is to suggest that more Africans *should* be dying—in a normative rather than a descriptive sense. It exposes the expectation that if the world suffers, then Africa must suffer more.

We can collectively learn from the questions we ask, but questions that distract from useful or meaningful comparisons dominate the current moment. Knowledge-making is about grappling with useful questions—those that move humanity toward greater understanding of our shared circumstances. "Why aren't more Africans dying of COVID-19?", like so many questions about Africa, fails to illuminate.

Some of the false frames on the question are obvious: "Africa" is a geographical construct that serves specific social and political functions, but it does not accurately represent the variation and complexity of the second-largest continent on earth. Regarding COVID-19, differences abound. In East Africa, where I live, countries like Tanzania barely measured its spread until July 2021; in Kenya and Uganda, the methods used to count cases changed constantly and widespread testing capacity was lacking; Ethiopia, Sudan and Somalia navigated the pandemic under complex political situations. Every country is different, and "Africa" is a useless analytical construct.

The word "more" also presents a problem. The reader might wonder: "more" in comparison to what? Predictions that were made about the trajectory of the disease? African experts, like the WHO Africa office, have conceded that the predictions were based on the assumption that African governments would not act in the early days of the pandemic. Yet, they did act and drastic measures were taken. Several African countries also made masks mandatory earlier in the trajectory of the pandemic than many countries elsewhere. So, the underlying false presumption—that African societies would do nothing—was confounded.

"More" also suggests a loaded comparison: because the coronavirus has had a devastating effect in Europe, North America, South America and, indeed, parts of Asia, Africa could not have been spared. Perhaps the long shadow that Western imperialism still casts on the continent encourages the lazy tendency to view Africa through the lens of the United States and Europe's experience, to believe that Africa's trajectory must either mimic the West, as its logical extension, or fail on all the counts where the West succeeds, as its opposite and antithesis. So, it bears stating: Africa is not the anti-Europe or the anti-USA.

If useful questions avoid careless and empty comparisons, what should we be asking instead?

One useful question would flip the gaze back at Europe and North America: why have so many people there died of the novel coronavirus? In its 25 September 2020 briefing, the WHO's Africa office hinted at structural issues that have made the virus spread faster among vulnerable populations in those regions, raising many questions that should demand political action in coming years. First, families in the West and increasingly in the East increasingly place elderly relatives in nursing homes. We should ask why societies—both capitalist and nominally communist like China—increasingly cannot sustain multigenerational families with complimentary roles for all members. Should we revisit the social and labour arrangements that make it impossible for families to provide substantive care for older relatives within the family network, that make out-sourcing care necessary?

Second, do the ways in which our cities are structured create vulnerabilities? The United Nations estimates that by 2050, more than two-thirds of the world's population will be living in urban areas, compared to just over half today. The most urbanised regions are in the West (82% of people in North America, 81% in South America, 74% in Europe); Africa, by contrast, is still mostly rural, with only around 43 per cent of its population living in urban areas.[1] Yet, the structure of our metropolises is part of the reason why COVID-19 has torn through many of the world's wealthier countries. The problem is not just the human density of cities, but also the pressure to circulate constantly, to enter and leave multiple spaces—the office, the gym, the supermarket, the nail salon, the barber—as a marker of urban vitality and as a way of promoting the economic health of the whole country. Why don't our urban economies allow us to stay still? We also have to think about the exploited underclass that makes city life possible in so many of the larger metropolises—the migrant workers of New York, London and Singapore who are critical to local economies but locked out of quality healthcare. And we will have to acknowledge that cities such as Auckland or Barcelona, which provided not just healthcare but also financial support to everyone, regardless of their national origin, fared better during the pandemic than those where unequal access is structural.

To ask why the coronavirus is having one trajectory in one place and not another can be a useful comparison if it takes into account policy measures, local contexts, the community response and the evolving state of knowledge about the disease. The earliest predictions about the trajectory of COVID-19 in Africa were dire, painting a worst-case scenario so that people would act urgently. People acted, and in most African countries, senior policy officials didn't lose time casting doubt on the severity of the disease or debating the usefulness of masks—the tool that has proven the single most useful in stemming the spread of the disease—in the same way as they did in the UK or United States. The then director of the Centers for Disease Control and Prevention in the US, Dr Robert R. Redfield, stated in September 2020 that masks would likely be more effective in controlling the coronavirus for the foreseeable future than a vaccine. So, why did Americans argue incessantly about them? What is it about the way that societies evolved in the US and parts of Europe that has allowed politics to have an outsized impact on public health? That is a better question. Good questions don't ask why more Africans aren't dying; they explore what officials did right and wrong and what we can learn from it.

Other useful comparisons might look at the trajectory of COVID-19 in specific African countries alongside its path in countries with similar economies and climates. For example, why was Ecuador devastated by COVID-19 (see Chapter 1), but Kenya experienced a slower progression of the disease? To what extent does this reflect the fact that in April 2020, Kenya made masks mandatory in public places and closed schools, religious buildings and other places where large numbers of people might gather? While some people argue that the numbers can't be trusted because of the differences in testing regimes, comparing the trajectories of similar countries is not useless; we can ask questions about the key moments of change. At what point did the graphs of deaths and cases change direction, if at all, and why?

Useful questions may lead us to confront just how loaded our daily discourse about this pandemic is. If the trajectory of COVID-19 in most African countries is consistent with that of other countries that took early action to flatten the curve, many European and North American nations would be forced to confront the reality that their politics is broken and their policy-making is not always the best. Useful questions interrogate the current global order, challenging normative ideas about how neoliberal states must be structured.

The art of asking useful questions demands that we push past superficial description to consider what drives each society forward. Useful questions set aside presumptions and biases about how the world must work and invite us to start imagining alternatives. Useful questions see that societies are more than just economies that must grow indefinitely regardless of how many people die in the process. And those questions will be invaluable in reconstructing society in the wake of COVID-19.

When we replace closed-ended presumptions about how the world *must* work with considerations about how the world *could* work, suddenly the future looks less set in stone and more of a consequence of collective choice.

11

DEATH AND FUNERAL ANNOUNCEMENTS

Newspapers in the UK have a section for notices where people can buy space to announce births, deaths, weddings and baptisms. Because Kenya is a former British colony, our newspapers have a similar tradition. Our oldest newspaper that's still in print, today known as *The Standard*, was founded in 1902. Sometimes, when I'm writing something that draws heavily on history, I go to the Kenya National Archives in Nairobi or the National Library at Community-Upper Hill in the same city and flip through pages of *The Standard*, not just to understand the thing I'm researching, but to help me imagine what the country was like at that time.

I find it interesting that in Kenya we no longer do birth, wedding or baptism announcements. We stopped sharing our good news with each other and now just share the bad. The only announcements that survive in Kenya are for deaths and funerals, which families of all incomes still put out religiously. Sometimes we also get death anniversary announcements as the family commemorates the passing of a loved one. Death is a major thing in our communities. The fact that we've held on to this banal practice gives you an idea of how our many cultures view death and death rites.

It also means that death and funeral announcements become an important forensic research tool when trying to put together the story of a moment or an event. For example, on 15 January 2016, Kenyan soldiers deployed in Somalia as part of the African Union Mission to Somalia (AMISOM) to stabilise this country and confront the Al-Shabaab terrorist group were attacked. Their camp was completely overrun by the militants. But the Kenyan government refused to confirm the size and scale of the killings on the basis of "national security".[1] That alone was a sure-fire indicator that something had gone terribly wrong at the El Adde military base. Suspicions were confirmed when the death and funeral announcements for various young soldiers started to appear in the newspapers, page after page of young men who had recently served in the army, mostly from the North Eastern Province, who had somehow all died at around the same time. The government has never given an official death toll for El Adde, but the Somalian prime minister Hassan Sheikh Mohamud was quoted as saying at least 180 were confirmed dead.[2]

I think about El Adde a lot when I read articles about the mystery of low COVID-19 death rates in Africa. Two years into the pandemic, on 22 March 2022, *The New York Times* published an article called "Trying to Solve a Covid Mystery: Africa's Low Death Rates".[3] *Nature* published an article referencing a study (which had not been peer reviewed) which claimed that 90 per cent of the people tested at a morgue in Lusaka, the capital of Zambia, tested positive for COVID-19.[4] There are three characters or voices in the article: a US-based global health specialist who says that there is an enormous undercounting of death in Lusaka; a South African epidemiologist who states that most of the people tested in their separate study were asymptomatic and soon recovered; and an Ethiopian physiologist who indicates that while the claim of undercounting cannot be discounted, "our experience is people get infected with the virus, are asymptomatic or have mild symptoms, and recover". Having COVID-19 doesn't mean dying from COVID-19. I'm uneasy with the binary that so much of this reporting is leaning towards—that one truth precludes the other. I think about the death and funeral announcements, and I wonder if the truth is not closer to the middle. We know that African governments have been unable to test at the level of wealthier countries. But does that then automatically mean that there is a wave of secret death that cannot be perceived, or worse, is being actively hidden?

During the worst of HIV/AIDS, we also had a moment when it was impossible to keep track of the number of people who had died or were dying. Even the official numbers of deaths for HIV/AIDS were ultimately estimates. In 2018, the National AIDS Control Council found that four of the Kenya's forty-seven counties had double digit HIV prevalence.[5] All four were in the western part of the country. This is where my family is from, and we knew that the situation was bad because funerals are a big deal in our community. During the worst of the HIV/AIDS pandemic, it felt like we were going to a funeral every other week. When people are dying at staggering rates, you don't need an official number to tell you that something has gone wrong. You can see it in the speed at which the death rites are repeated.

I think about the death and funeral announcements a lot when I read all these stories about secret deaths in Africa. The idea that we simply throw our dead into the ground and forget about them doesn't correspond to the culture that I know. Granted, this culture does not represent the whole continent, but I think this is an important counterargument. There seems to be a misguided belief that because many of us in Africa live in communities where we do not kiss or hold hands in public—that because our love is less performative than it is in the West—that, some-how, we love less? This is an exceptionally racist view. To love is the most fundamental part of what it means to be human. And if you paid attention, you would see that our death rites reflect a deep culture of care and love for those closest to us. We do not simply throw our dead into the ground and forget about them.

With this in mind, many of us were paying attention to the death and funeral announcements during the COVID-19 pandemic. We knew that the government was misrepresenting the number of people who had died. We knew that there was a delib-erate effort to under-test because the government just wouldn't spend the money needed on public health. We knew that as hos-pitals started to fill up, we could no longer get treatment for sim-pler illnesses. We knew that if death started to happen at scale, we would see an uptick in the number of death and funeral announce-ments in the newspapers for people who died "after a short ill-ness". It wouldn't be an exact count, but it would be a sample that could give us a sense of how bad the pandemic was going.

I never ran the numbers on it. I can only tell you, anecdotally, that the newspapers did not become an endless litany of death and funeral announcements. I can only tell you that our death rites may not look like yours, but we do not simply throw our dead into the ground and forget about them. I think about how these death and funeral announcements have persisted through economic collapse and political upheaval, and I am reminded that care and love find different forms of expression in different soci-eties. I do believe that at some level there is more death than the official numbers will tell us, because the government simply did not want to count. But I can also tell you that if death was hap-pening at the scale that some of these articles about COVID-19 in Africa suggested, we would have noticed.

We do not simply throw our dead into the ground and forget about them.

12

DISPOSABLE PEOPLE

People kept creating, expanding and adapting the labels to give us a shorthand to describe what we were seeing. They kept throwing labels around as if categorising people and then using those categories to label the disease would help us get to grips with everything faster. The same thing had happened years before in deciding that HIV/AIDS was first "a gay disease", then an "African disease". Once it became "Those People's Problem", then there was no need for wealthy, heterosexual Westerners to remain vigilant. "As long as *we* avoid the risk of contagion from *them*, then we will be fine and everything will be normal." So, we scrambled for labels to help the mind contain the threat of the coronavirus so that we could figure out how to respond to it.

First, it was the Wuhan virus, then it was the Chinese virus, and, for a few moments, it was a broadly Asian virus, because some people couldn't even be bothered to make any fine distinctions—they just wanted a "them" to their "us" so they knew who they needed to hate and avoid. Then it became a disease of travellers, so there was a scramble to figure out which borders needed to be closed and which borders had to stay open. It was okay to ban travellers from Asia entirely, but when it came to banning travellers from wealthy white countries, most nations vacillated and hedged, even when the worst of the pandemic was happening in Europe and the USA. And then doctors and nurses started dying at alarming rates, and it quickly became clear that no amount of labelling would hermetically seal us off from this new disease. Whatever categories we established and whatever walls we put around them would be insufficient to keep the disease at bay.

In the process of scrambling to delineate these boundaries, something even more sinister started to happen. We inadvertently started creating groups of people for whom death would be a tolerable outcome. Not that these groups didn't exist before: there are entire families of diseases that kill millions around the world and for which there is no research into or investment in understanding or preventing them, because the people dying are poor, or not-white. Some of them are called Neglected Tropical Diseases. Every year, up to 400 million people contract dengue fever and around 40,000 die from the disease.[1] And the most deadly disease in the world by a great distance is malaria, which doesn't qualify as a neglected disease, but certainly does not receive nearly as much research funding as COVID-19 has received since it was discovered in 2019. The World Health Organization estimates that 627,000 people died of malaria in 2020—96 per cent of these deaths were in Africa and 80 per cent of them were children.[2] The idea of a double standard for providing healthcare is not in itself novel.

I think what was truly different this time around was that the circle of who was worth keeping alive was so small. As the disease progressed, it was as if new categories of disposable people were being created every day. Doctors and nurses died because governments that would spend billions on their militaries and police services suddenly could not find the money for personal protective equipment (PPE).[3] And this trend was one of the few that was consistent all over the world. After years of deprioritising public health, most countries simply did not have the agility to protect healthcare workers.[4] Teachers were also forced to return to the classroom with few modifications to their working environment. Sure, some of us got to work from home or make alternative arrangements, but for so many people who provide the crucial services that make our societies tick, there were simply no concessions.

In 2020, after the doctors and nurses, it was elderly people, and particularly those living in long-term care homes, who were hit the hardest. A June 2020 study found that in Canada, residents of long-term care homes accounted for more than 80 per cent of the country's COVID-19 deaths during the first few months of the pandemic, compared to an average of 38 per cent across other Organisation for Economic Co-operation and Development (OECD) countries.[5] By March 2021, 8 per cent of all the people living in long-term care facilities in the US had died of COVID-19.[6] In fact, The COVID Tracking Project, which produced this data, believes that it was a gross undercount, and argues that "long-term-care facility deaths made up over a third of all US deaths".[7] In all of the countries that were collecting information, until the widespread use of vaccination, there was a strong correlation between living in a long-term care home and death from COVID-19.[8] Some countries responded by locking the elderly away from younger family members, based in part on the narrative that young people were not getting as sick as older people. But only when vaccines became widely available did the momentum of death in elderly care homes slow down.

Perhaps as chilling as the experience of watching so many elderly people die in such isolation was the reaction of some governments to this widespread death. It was almost as if the pandemic made older people and chronically ill people disposable overnight. The Swedish case is probably the best known because it seemed like a new level of dystopia in an already difficult time. More than 70 per cent of Sweden's COVID-19 deaths up to May 2020 were in elderly care homes.[9] Sweden's pandemic strategy was to remain as close to "normal" as possible, eschewing masks and social-distancing and the myriad other measures that other countries elsewhere put in place to slow down the disease.[10] The argument was that because COVID-19 was primarily devastating to older people and people with comorbidities, it simply wasn't worth disrupting the majority's lives in an effort to protect the more vulnerable. The government committed to "ring-fencing" the elderly and then allowing everyone else to carry on as normal. But eventually, the Swedish government had to concede that the plan had failed and had led to an unnecessary loss of life because elderly care homes did not have the capacity to provide the protection that the system presumed.[11]

Children were not spared this narrative of disposability, either. At first, almost all children across the world were withdrawn from school, but in many countries, the infection numbers just kept going up, and so the children were sent back to the classroom. The alternative sounds much worse though. In Uganda, children were kept out of school for almost two years because of the pandemic on the promise that they would be learning online. But the online learning did not materialise and many simply dropped out. Research on vaccinating children also came slowly, and so children were literally being thrown back into the riskiest context—extended periods indoors in crowded conditions and with poor ventilation—without the main defence that we have developed against the disease. We simply had to return to "normal" regardless of the potential cost.

And people with disabilities and with comorbidities? Well, they were routinely completely forgotten or even actively placed in harm's way. A 2020 paper published by the American

Sociological Association catalogued some of the way people with disabilities were actively singled out as being expendable in the context of the pandemic.[12] During a protest against lockdowns in Tennessee in April 2020, one protester held up a sign reading "Sacrifice the weak—Reopen TN". A report from the UK Office for National Statistics found that between 24 January and 30 November 2020, the risk of death from COVID-19 in England was 3.1 times higher for men with significant disabilities and 3.5 times higher for women with significant disabilities than those without disabilities.[13] And yet the specific risks facing people with disabilities were similarly ignored all over the world. Very few countries explicitly put in place policies as simple as making sure that information about COVID-19 was available in multiple formats.[14]

You hope that one of the things that people have learnt through this experience of the pandemic is that capitalism can make any one of us disposable at any time, depending on the exigencies of the moment. You hope that people notice and condemn the argument that keeping the machine going was a more important outcome than providing care for the most vulnerable. But based on the way policymaking continues to steamroll over the concerns of people who don't fit capitalism's description of productivity, it seems we haven't fully appreciated the lesson. Of course, empathy demands that we provide for each other in our communities, not just because one day we might need it, but because it's the right thing to do. But even in that context, the lack of solidarity with these groups has been shocking and a terrifying window into the paradigms of disposability that have taken root worldwide.

Fewer and fewer of us can live the way our grandparents or even our parents did, and we are certainly not going to be able to grow old the way they did. This is a universal truth. In agrarian societies, the industrialisation of agriculture means that there are fewer and fewer of us who are working the land and living in communities that can provide the kind of multigenerational elderly care we had in the past. And urbanisation has unleashed a slew of unprecedented problems that the pandemic just made more serious. Actual retirement into a life of relaxation is a myth. We are living longer and working longer, but that also means more years of sustained care. We are unable to be present for our seniors the way they were for theirs, because capitalism demands our constant attention. Multigenerational households are shrinking because more of us are having to move away from home to find meaningful work.

For some people, this isn't necessarily a universally bad thing. If you're a woman who comes from a traditionally patriarchal society, or if you are LGBTQ+ person in a homophobic community, life in the city offers a measure of freedom and the chance to build your chosen family. But human beings are fundamentally social beings, and the ideal world would obviously be one in which everyone is able to find love and acceptance within the family they have.

Watching elderly people in care homes first get separated from their families and then die because of policy failures was a chilling stage in the pandemic. The assumption was, in many countries, that the main thing we needed to do to address the disease was to protect the working-aged people because children and the elderly were surplus to the needs of the system—providing labour, buying and paying for things. The deaths in the elderly care homes were just one of the perverse outcomes of this argument. If you think about it, though, we all get born, but we only grow old if we are lucky. And yet modernity fetishises youth and treats older people with so much disdain. It showed us that in this system we have built, we are all valued for our labour, and perhaps our beauty, but not much else. And not all youth, because children were also getting the short end of the stick. Children were forced to go back to school while the pandemic raged because their parents needed to go back to work. Many children died of COVID-19, and today it is obvious that the idea that children do not get seriously ill from the virus is simply untrue.

There aren't that many long-term care facilities for the elderly in Kenya. The Catholic Church runs one or two primarily to serve members of religious congregations who might not have family to care for them in their senior years. Two of the last three archbishops of Nairobi died at one such facility. Most people as they get older expect to live with extended family, particularly relatives in rural areas who might not have had as much chance at the relentless capitalist lifestyle of urban areas. Multigenerational living is normal in rural areas and present, but less common, in urban contexts, with older family members providing holiday or seasonal care for younger family members. It's also worth pointing out that women's labour is a big part of what makes these systems work. Usually, a younger female relative brought in from a poorer part of the family is conscripted to do the care work, often unpaid or poorly paid. The system that privileges keeping elderly parents close to home succeeds on the back of a lot of women's labour.

But older relatives also contribute to the home. The point of closing the generational loop was that grandparents could provide the social education that young people needed while the adults went off to labour. In peri-urban contexts, it is still the case that grandparents will take children for vacations or during holiday periods, but as people are having children older, it also means that people are becoming grandparents older, and at some point grandparents will not be able to keep up with the needs of a three-year-old. Maybe the future is in the beautiful stories coming out of intergenerational care homes that are both nurseries and facilities for older people, allowing caseworkers to focus on care and younger children to learn from their elders. Supporters say it fosters trust between the different generations.[15]

As more and more of us turn to the cities, we will increasingly have to contend with the new reality of growing old without the structures that our grandparents had to keep them safe. More of us will end up in elderly care homes and dependent on non-family members to help us during these vulnerable years. It's scary to think what the next pandemic will look like if we don't figure out how to help people age, well supported and in dignity. It's scary to think that this momentum towards city life is creating entirely new categories of disposable people, as we haven't figured out what to do when so many of us living so close together get sick.

13

VOCABULARIES

There are all these new words to learn just to figure out how to survive.

Comorbidity: an underlying condition conspiring with a new illness to cause even greater harm. Before 2020, I had no idea what a comorbidity was. Morbid comes from the Latin word *morbidus*, which means diseased. A comorbidity is like a co-wife or a co-husband. A disease working alongside another disease, sharing the labour of destroying the body from within.

One article in the BBC breaks down why this fixation with comorbidities was so unhelpful.[1] Because the reason why so many people with comorbidities were dying wasn't just because the conditions were conspiring to kill. It was because doctors and nurses—overworked, underpaid and overwhelmed by the incoming wave of grave illness—were having to make difficult decisions every day about where to send the resources that they had. Who should get the limited amount of oxygen that could be found in the hospital? The eighty-year-old grandmother who is loved and wanted, but whose frail body might not properly respond to the steroids required to bring a person off the ventilator? The person who arrived at the hospital first, even though they are already so far gone in the trajectory of infection that it would take a miracle to bring them back?

Health policymakers call it catastrophe medicine. The context of catastrophe medicine is different from practicing medicine in ordinary times, and tough choices must be made. The coronavirus pandemic put an enormous burden on these doctors and nurses to decide who to save based on who the science says can be saved. It weighed so heavily on so many of them, having to deny people treatment, not because it cannot work but because it might not work. It forced these medical professionals into making assessments that almost contravened the vow they made to protect human life: first do no harm. It put more strain on all the frontline workers who were already doing more every day than they signed up for.

The contemporary meaning of morbid is "characterised by an abnormal and unhealthy interest in disturbing and unpleasant subjects, especially death and disease". And so, the practice of medicine during the pandemic has itself become morbid, forced into a harmful obsession with death and disease because there was so very little room for things like life, hope and care. Operating at the precipice of community and what it meant to belong to one, so many of us were forced to become morbid—constantly calculating, even during routine tasks, what implications they would have for our likelihood of getting sick, or even dying.

We started to memorise comorbidities, as if knowing that they exist would be an extra layer of protection. They started to seep into ordinary conversations in which people would actively try to negotiate with the virus within them: "I can do this because I don't have that"; "this couldn't happen to me because I don't have that". But some of the logic began to fray almost immediately. It is no longer possible to argue that children do not get COVID-19. It is no longer possible to say that it is just a disease of the elderly. And with Long COVID, it is no longer possible to state that death is the only thing to fear. We are still learning which of the factors that come to mind are actual comorbidities and which are simply coincidences. This is the nature of science and research.

I feel the morbidity settle into my own conscience. So many of my friends are doctors and nurses, and I am heartbroken by the idea that they might be forced to make these decisions themselves. According to a July 2020 study, Kenya had only 537 Intensive Care Unit (ICU) beds for a nation of roughly 48 million people.[2] Many of these beds are in private hospitals that are completely out of reach for ordinary people. The pandemic is a moment that should have invited major and rapid investment into the health system, but it hasn't happened because the politics is toxic and poisoning everything around it. In the early months of the pandemic, I ran into a friend of mine who is a doctor in the city's health system, but also a policymaker. We were masked and distanced, but on leaving sneaked in an illicit hug because he was so tired: tired of arguing for PPE, tired of fighting for resources to make the hospitals work better, tired of the long hours at work before going home at the end of the day to look at his own partner and children and say, "I don't know what's coming next".

Comorbidities at scale: underlying weaknesses or vulnerabilities that work together to intensify the impact of the pandemic on our collective ability to survive. Corruption, of course, was one, but also racism, ableism and a host of other "-isms" which imply an innate inability to empathise with or see other people as fully human and therefore worthy of our concern. There were also other diseases that weighed down social and economic systems because the people who ran them were unable to act with the urgency and focus that is needed to avoid widespread disaster. There were preconfigured injustices that narrowed down our path to action so that we did not focus on what it was right to do, but only on what the system dictated could be done.

What is the opposite of a comorbidity, I wonder? In language-learning, an easy way to make peace with new vocabulary is to memorise words in pairs: to learn what it is and what it is not at the same time so we can easily express presence or absence. What word do we have for things that work together to help or to heal a person from an illness that they encounter? I don't think there is one. There are clumsy formulations that always end up at the same place. "Mitigating factors", comes to mind. There don't seem to be enough mitigating factors to memorise, only comorbidities that conspired to steal our loved ones from us.

14

THE FEARS OF THE OTHER

The government will not do anything.

The police/the army/the solders are going to kill us before this disease does.

No one in the government knows what they are talking about.

Everyone in the government knows more than they are letting on.

No one is coming to help us.

No one is seeing the many ways we are helping each other and ourselves.

The medicine is going to make us sick.

We are being experimented on with things that have not been tested.

We cannot make the medicine we need to keep ourselves safe.

There will not be any medicine left for us.

We will not be able to feed our children if everything is locked down.

We will not be able to feed ourselves if we cannot even feed our children.

We have too many other equally—if not more important—things to worry about.

This disease is like that other one that killed so many people.

They will use up all the medicine and leave nothing on the table for us.

They are waiting for this to become an "African disease" so that *they* can say we brought it on ourselves.

They are not giving us the same medicine that they are using over there.

They are not telling us everything about this pandemic.

NORMAL

15

OMICRON

In February 2021, I took a socially distanced trip across Western Kenya, driving solo along some of the most beautiful country roads and visiting the national parks outside the country's tourist circuit. In many of these places, I was the only visitor, the park rangers having grown accustomed to the silences created by the pandemic. One of these parks is the Kakamega Forest National Reserve, the last remaining stretch of rainforest in Kenya which, before intense human activity, was once part of the mighty Congo rainforest system. The rainforest is home to several rare species of birds, butterflies and apes. Kenya's game reserves, as opposed to game parks, are also unique because they allow human activity. You can harvest fruit and graze cattle in the reserves, but you are not allowed to live there. So, it was unusual but not entirely unexpected to find three young boys in the Kakamega Forest under an improvised canopy of broad leaves, singing and making percussion with empty plastic containers and sticks. They were using the age-old methods of harvesting termites from a large termite mound. It was a fantastic thing to witness, and I made a recording and shared it on my social media. One of my friends saw the video and sent me a private message, asking me more about what I had seen. As long as I'd known her, she had always been one of the most curious and passionate people I had ever met, so this didn't surprise me too much. We had a great but brief conversation and I promised to tell her more about it when we saw each other after the lockdown ended.

We never got to have that conversation because two weeks after we spoke, in March 2021, she had died from COVID-19. Indeed, she had been messaging me while in hospital receiving treatment for it. I like to think that I'm the kind of person who has taken COVID-19 seriously from the beginning, but there is something about losing someone who you literally just spoke to in such an unexpected manner that makes things even more real and urgent. This was the reality of the coronavirus for so many people. One day the people you loved were here and then moments later they were gone.

In April of that year, the Kenyan government had announced that it had no intention to vaccinate its population under the age of fifty. I would not be receiving a vaccine in Kenya. At the same time, many of the professional conversations that help keep the electricity on at my house were starting up again in Europe and North America, and there was an assumption that I would participate in person. By May 2021, it became clear that I was going to have to travel again. It was a strange season, being in all these conversations with supposed colleagues and "partners" gushing effusively about how vaccines had fixed everything and how thrilled they were to be returning to normal now that the pandemic was finally over. Time and time again, finding myself the only African on these calls, I had to interrupt and say, "that sounds nice, but we don't have any vaccines and there doesn't seem to be any pathway to getting them here any time soon". At least some of these folks had the decency to be embarrassed, but it was one of those personal experiences that test the concept of "solidarity", what it means to be among people who study African politics or history as an abstract idea but struggle to comprehend the lives of African people.

So, I made a plan. I gathered together a bit of money, messaged a friend in the US and asked if I could sleep on their sofa, and used my tourist visa to go and get one of those millions of doses of vaccines that they were eventually going to throw away instead of letting us have them. I have no regrets about that decision. But the injustice of the whole thing left a sour taste in my mouth that has never really gone away. It is a strange thing, to be having theoretical conversations about inequality one week and in the next, to be standing in line, watching a young Spanish-speaking man nervously ask the nurse if his father needed ID in order to get vaccinated. It was a strange experience to have to keep reminding people that there are limits to the privilege that unites those who have been able to maintain a steady income and relative safety through this period of unprecedented upheaval, and that some of us, simply by virtue of our identities, were constantly on the wrong side of these limits.

There are so many layers of injustice that the COVID-19 pandemic has made rawer and more urgent. For a long time, perhaps since the end of the Cold War in the 1990s, the lines between real and aspirational values of human and national relations have been blurred. It hasn't always been clear when speaking about the way we relate or expect to relate to each other if we're talking about things as they are or things as we want them to be. For those of us who came of age after the Cold War, it was as if we inherited a promise. The promise was that if we championed certain values of freedom, democracy, justice and more, then we would never have to live through some of the horrors that our predecessors had endured in brutal world wars, widespread devastating disease and unprecedented economic collapse. There had been a before, and we had all learnt from it, and if we just embraced these values and followed this path, then all would be well for us in future.

There aren't that many people left who embrace this line of thinking. Even Francis Fukuyama, who made a name for himself with his theory about how the end of the Cold War signalled the end of history, has renounced the position. He once argued that without major ideological conflicts, human beings would now focus all their energies on attaining his version of liberal ideals. Today, even he concedes that what we were living through may have been the calm before the storm.

And what a storm it is. The guns and bombs have gotten bigger and more elaborate, and now the wars are worse than they have ever been. Economies are collapsing and democracies are disintegrating into authoritarian habits. And then there are new overarching threats like climate change and this pandemic that make it all too clear that we need to have another conversation about what these values represent, and what it means to work together to achieve them. It's not so much that the values themselves have changed—democracy, justice and equality are still objectively good things that everyone should aspire to and work towards. But it is increasingly clear that there's a moral relativism embedded in what version of democracy some people get and what version others are offered. There hasn't been an honest reckoning with the "-isms" that flow through our societies, and that makes both the values and the journey towards achieving them less clear.

The pandemic has been a focal point for too many of these "-isms". Racism, ableism, nationalism in its most pejorative sense, and classism, especially, have stood in the way of a truly global response. Too many people showed the hollowness of their politics of solidarity, and it made too many others question the point of having these values in the first place. It didn't have to be this way. This could have been a moment to make a statement about how much has changed since the world last fell apart with the HIV/AIDS pandemic. Instead, it was a reminder that true change and true transformation require intent. But an intent to be better than the past is alarmingly missing from many of those who wield power.

The greed and selfishness of the first year of the pandemic was disturbing enough, but even when vaccines emerged and there was a moment to reset within the narrow context of COVID-19, the people with power still refused to be better. The emergence of the Omicron variant in late November 2021 seems to have brought out the worst in the West, and, indeed, in powerful countries the world over, particularly in the nasty reaction to the possibility that a variant may have emerged from Africa. Since the initial jabs were rolled out, some critics of their uneven distribution argued that it was important to provide vaccines to Africa because without them, the disease would continue to evolve and a new variant would surely soon emerge. Scientifically, it's the correct argument. But it seems to have been interpreted as meaning it was only a matter of time before a deadly variant emerged from Africa, and that countries should be on standby to protect themselves from African people when that day finally came.

You see proof of this in the way countries responded to the discovery of Omicron. In late November 2021, Dr Sikhulile Moyo, a Zimbabwean virologist at the Botswana–Harvard HIV Reference Laboratory (BHHRL), noticed an unusual sequence of genes in a COVID-19 sample that he and his team had been investigating, and notified the authorities (as was the required protocol).[1] Crucially, the samples were taken from diplomats who had been tested on entering Botswana, and whose previous travel included into and out of Europe. Almost simultaneously, researchers at South Africa's Lancet Laboratories in Pretoria made a similar discovery in a COVID-19 sample they had taken.[2] The virus had mutated in alarming and unprecedented ways, with nearly fifty genetic modifications—the most mutations of any COVID-19 variant. Once again, these scientists shared this information with the relevant authorities and, in December 2021, the WHO declared Omicron a variant of concern.

No previous discoveries of new variants were treated with as much acrimony as this one; no other sequence of events served to remind African people that we were not among the number when people talked about "the world". Instead of receiving acknowledgement for the scientific labour that had gone into discovering the new variant, African countries were punished with extreme travel bans. Some countries like Japan and Israel put in place universal travel bans. Others like the US and the UK prohibited travellers from South Africa, Namibia, Zimbabwe, Botswana, Mozambique, Malawi, Zambia, Lesotho and Eswatini, with the UK adding Angola to that list unless the traveller was a returning resident.[3] The EU suspended travel from southern Africa, with then German health minister Jens Spahn arguing that "The last thing we need is to bring in a new variant that will cause even more problems", while failing to acknowledge how variants from Europe had caused so many problems elsewhere.[4] Countries like Argentina made quarantine mandatory for anyone who had been on the African continent within the previous fourteen days, but not anyone who had been in Europe or North America.

How do you make sense of that? That despite warnings about the potential of new variants emerging in unvaccinated populations, many of these countries were unwilling to act, but when a possible new variant did emerge, they were so quick to implement harsh and unprecedented bans against an entire continent? How do you make sense of this reluctance to take simple measures to prevent a specific outcome and then this disproportionate reaction when that outcome *possibly* comes to pass?

The racism at the heart of these decisions was quickly evident, as the scientists in Botswana confirmed that the samples in which the new mutations had been detected had come from Europe. Days later, scientists in Germany and the Czech Republic confirmed that Omicron had been detected in people with no history of travel to southern Africa.[5] In December, Dutch authorities confirmed that the strain had been present in samples taken in the Netherlands before the it had been discovered in South Africa.[6] The same sequence of events would take place in the US, although it wouldn't be until January that the country would ease travel restrictions against southern Africa. Omicron did not emerge in southern Africa—it was merely detected there—but African countries were being punished for doing the world a great favour in pointing out a new variant of concern that could evade the protection given by available vaccines.

It's this itchiness to watch African countries fail that really gnaws at me. Where was the global solidarity when people were begging for medicine? It's this underlying heart of darkness fallacy that claims contagion and deadly disease only travel in one direction. Where was this alarm when the risk was of people from Europe and North America bringing disease to Africa? Where was this abundance of caution when we were warning that an outbreak might completely cripple our public health systems? It's this quickness with which we are stigmatised and marginalised that tells a terrifying story about how hollow the promises of some of these liberal values are. Why are there concerns about open borders in southern Africa when Europe's borders are in fact the most open in the world?

The power holders in the current world order seem to only comprehend Africa as a problem that requires their pity, and not as a place where people live. So, they unsee the rigorous science and labour—the contributions that African people are making towards addressing this universal challenge—but are quick to overreact when there is even the slightest possibility of trouble emerging from the continent. Africa must just have been lucky to have avoided a serious outbreak so far, the story goes; it has nothing to do with the efforts that African people are putting towards understanding, confronting and containing the spread of disease. Africa, in this imagination, is not a place where people do things. It is merely a place where bad things happen.

Omicron did indeed go on to be a problem in Europe and North America, mostly because, while countries were banning travellers from Africa, the disease was spreading rapidly at home. "It's impossible", says one of the characters in Camus' *The Plague*, "everyone knows it [the plague] has vanished from the West." To which another character appends, "Yes, everyone knew that, except the dead."[7] That belief that contagion naturally belongs in one part of the world because a certain type of people live there? That's racist. That inability to comprehend the possibility that an outbreak could happen somewhere simply because of the identities of the people who live there? That's racist, too. And that racism leaves room for the kind of devastation that Omicron and its subvariants are still wreaking across Europe and North America, even in 2022. If we can't see a universal human risk for what it is in a moment like this, then when?

African countries have so much to teach the world about surviving pandemics. We are still clawing our way out of the last major pandemic—the HIV/AIDS pandemic of the 1990s. Too many of us lost people that we loved to this novel disease, but through the heartbreak, we learnt so much about what it takes to survive devastation at this scale. It is not a coincidence that so much of the public health infrastructure that has helped African countries navigate COVID-19 was until recently dedicated to addressing HIV/AIDS. The Botswana lab that did the first round of genetic sequencing that identified Omicron is a HIV/AIDS research lab. The community healthcare systems that developed public health messaging that went out to remote communities that rarely ever see a nurse, let alone a doctor, was developed to communicate the risks of HIV/AIDS easily and quickly in multiple languages to people of varying linguistic capacity. The solidarity systems that left us holding babies after their parents passed away can teach so much to the hundreds of thousands of children that have been orphaned by COVID-19. HIV/AIDS has devastated our communities, but we are not merely enduring it. We have learnt, we have worked together and we have built systems that made sense for our contexts in order to get through it.

No one was more passionate about Africa giving to the world than my friend, Lorna. She was deeply curious about everything about us; she was one of only two people who saw that video I shared and who asked to know more. When you were in her company, she inevitably made you feel like you were the most important person in the world. She loved us. That she died weeks before the first doses of COVID-19 vaccines arrived in Kenya will never not be heart-breaking to me, and I'm sure also to those who loved her more intimately. She was taken away from her family and her friends far too soon because too many people failed to see the Africa that she saw and loved—a place of possibility and joy that deserved more and better. Our loss is part of a bigger tapestry of loss woven by this pandemic: losses caused by greed and human inaction. Our loss is a reminder that these political choices have consequences at a human level. But Africans shouldn't have to be as singular and remarkable as Lorna to be exempted from the onerous consequences of global politics shaped by "-isms", instead of solidarity. We should be aspiring to do better for everyone simply because they are human. Because everyone we lose to the folly of not doing so is someone's Lorna.

16

THE NUMBERS ON THAT

When the pandemic started, the major concern was that the world's economy would collapse and it would lead to chaos. Instead, something more perverse seems to have happened. Those who had lots now have even more—far more than they actually need—and those who had nothing somehow have even less. The companies that manufacture vaccines are making record- breaking profits. The people who own them have become billionaires. What are we to make of a world in which people would deny others access to life-saving medicines because they want to make more money? What are we to conclude about a system that not only encourages but even celebrates this as a sign of progress?

Despite assertions that this pandemic would be a great equaliser, it has instead turned out to be an accelerator of inequality. The ten richest people in the world doubled their fortunes during the first two years of the pandemic, and yes, they are all men.[1] The wealth of US billionaires grew by 44 per cent between March 2020 and February 2021, or about US $1.3 trillion.[2] In Asia, there are twenty new pandemic billionaires, even though

140 million people fell into poverty.[3] Many of these new billionaires have made their fortunes by selling us the things that we needed to survive—vaccines, PPE, all kinds of medicine. There is something truly perverse about a system that rewards those who already have with more while so many people continue to suffer.

One billion in digits is 1,000,000,000. I think it's important to write these things out sometimes so that we all have a clear sense of what we are talking about. It's as if when we talk about the difference between a million and a billion we can flatten out the yawning gap between them because only one letter changes. Maybe it makes us feel like only one zero is added. But a billion is a million one thousand times over, and a multibillionaire is someone who has that many times. And some people increased their wealth by these factors merely in the three years that the rest of us were trying to stay two steps ahead of the virus. Not necessarily because of something that they did—if you think about it, they are merely one cog in a giant machine. What kind of world have we built when such things are not just normal but celebrated? When the measure of success becomes accumulation for the sake of accumulation, particularly while staring down a disaster?

The pandemic will go down in history as the largest transfer of wealth from the poor to the rich ever. In the US, around 20 million people lost their jobs as the virus hit. By UN estimates, global unemployment will rise to its highest levels in history, with over 200 million new cases, as a direct result of the pandemic. Women, who were already relatively more precariously employed, lost 5 per cent of all jobs in 2020, while men lost 3.9 per cent. Millions of migrant workers and day labourers were no longer able to work because of the brutally enforced shutdowns, bearing the brunt of the broken promise that lockdowns were a temporary measure designed to hold the outbreak back until a longer-term solution was found. Losing a job in itself can be a tremendous source of stress and anxiety, loss of face and self-worth. But in this capitalist world we have built, for many people, a job means access to healthcare, education, clean water and decent food. Yet, some people have emerged from this pandemic with far more than they need or could ever consume in millions of lifetimes.

Look at the fortunes of the various vaccine manufacturers. Different companies in different countries made vaccines, but one thing that unites them all is that at some point, they all received public funding—money that is taken from taxpayers and given to them—to advance their work. The product of such investments should therefore theoretically be made available for public good rather than for private profit. Moreover, the reason why these companies were able to develop mRNA-based vaccines so quickly was because taxpayer-funded research sequenced the coronavirus genome and made those findings available in peer-reviewed academic publications.[4] The development of mRNA jabs was not an individual eureka moment. It was the culmination of years of scientific inquiry supported by public funding.

Operation Warp Speed in the United States, for example, which accelerated the development of the Moderna vaccine, was a taxpayer-funded initiative.[5] What's more, the research that made that the vaccine of Swedish–British company AstraZeneca possible was done by the University of Oxford, and funded over several years by the European Commission and the UK government, as well as charitable organisations like the Wellcome Trust.[6] Without the University of Oxford, itself an academic institution that receives government funding in addition to tuition fees, there is no AstraZeneca COVID-19 vaccine. In January 2020, AstraZeneca was worth US $130 billion. By January 2022, its value had shot up to US $177 billion.

Moreover, around 2,000 South Africans took part in the global medical trials for the AstraZeneca vaccine, as did approximately 400 Kenyans.[7] The trials were mostly funded by the Wellcome Trust, but also required the collaboration of South African and Kenyan research institutes like the South Africa Medical Research Council's Vaccine and Infectious Diseases Analytics research Unit (VIDA) and the Kenya Medical Research Institute (KEMRI). This was not Alexander Fleming stumbling upon penicillin in his laboratory by himself. It was years of collaborative research across continents, funded by the public purse of multiple countries, with people from all over the world volunteering their bodies as the final site for testing whether the gamble would pay off.

So, the fact that all of AstraZeneca's profits are being distributed to a small coterie of shareholders really gets to the heart of the injustices of the current economic system. It's a giant straw sucking up the sacrifices and the contributions of various publics and turning them into a completely useless pile of unusable money for a handful of people. Unusable, because even if you tried your hardest, a single person cannot spend multiple billions of dollars in just one lifetime. Even if you bought one of everything that there is to buy in the world, you would still be left with billions more unspent. And this is what makes it a particularly futile transfer of wealth. The pursuit of fortune by a handful of people makes the world intolerably crueller; the concept of riches as a buffer against this cruelty compounds the irrationality. You create the problem and then use the problem as a way of solving the problem. And then you take whatever meagre solution this thing you created can offer the most vulnerable and siphon it towards people who don't need it, can't use it and really only want to have it because the option exists.

AstraZeneca, for all its flaws, isn't even the most problematic of the group. At the very least, the company made a commitment to sell the vaccine at below market price for as long as the pandemic phase of the outbreak lasted, although even that turned out to be a nebulous promise. Leaked conversations revealed that while the company was charging European countries US $2.15 per dose, it was charging South Africa US $5.25, or more than double.[8] "Market price" means nothing if it still results in those who can afford it least paying more for the drug than those who can afford it most—the pricing still then functions as a transfer of wealth from poor countries to wealthy countries, because the shareholders that will split the proceeds will likely pay taxes in those wealthy countries. But even that US $5.25 is nothing compared to Moderna charging the United States US $15 per dose and the EU an exorbitant US $18, for a vaccine that was also developed using public funds.

Moderna has its origins in postgraduate research conducted between 2005 and 2009 at Harvard University—a private educational institution that receives millions in public research funding from bodies like the National Institute of Health. Moderna was registered as a company in 2010. Within two years of its founding, the company had raised US $40 million in funding, making it what investors call a "unicorn", but for the first eleven years of its existence, it failed to turn a single dollar in profit.[9] In 2021, the company had only one commercial product: its mRNA vaccine against COVID-19. Yet, in the same year, the company announced eye-watering revenues of US $18.5 billion and profits of US $12.2 billion.[10]

Let's write that out in full again so that we don't lose sight of what we are talking about. In 2020, Moderna's net loss was US $747 million. They made *negative* US $747,000,000. In 2021, Moderna's profit was US $12.2 billion. They made US $12,200,000,000. And in that time, they only sold one product. Their COVID-19 vaccine. Too many people around the world will read this and think it is an inspirational story. Too many people will see these figures but not the fact that Moderna received funding from US taxpayers through the Biomedical

Advanced Research and Development Authority (BARDA) to complete the research that it needed to make a commercially viable vaccine.[11] The company also received another US $10 billion from the American government to allow it to expand its manufacturing capacity, complete its large-scale clinical trials and bring its vaccines to market. Once again, the myth that this vaccine was the sole endeavour of an individual working only using their private resources and stumbling upon a vaccine completely by chance simply does not hold. The Moderna vaccine was a product of public funding, rooted in research conducted within a university that also receives significant amount of public funding. So, allowing the proceeds from that research to remain purely in a commercial company is not only absurd, but it fundamentally functions as a transfer of wealth.

The same pattern repeats with just about all the vaccines produced in Europe and North America. The Pfizer half of Pfizer–BioNTech insist that they did not receive any public funding, but the BioNTech half received at least €375 million from the German government and another €100 million in debt financing from the EU.[12] Russia's Sputnik vaccine, by far the most expensive vaccine of the European options, is an overt government project, supported by the Ministry of Health and with its research and distribution funded by the Russian Direct Investment Fund.[13]

Contrast this with Cuba's vaccination programme. According to the journal *Nature*, despite the weight of the US embargo on trade with the tiny island, the Cuban government supported the development of at least three vaccine candidates, one of which, Sobreana 02, is more than 90 per cent effective against symptomatic COVID-19.[14] Cuba's vaccination programme has barely received the international attention it deserves because of global geopolitics, but it seems to be paying off, and the institute developing the jabs has volunteered to make its technology as widely available as possible, particularly to poor countries. Cuba has administered one of the most effective COVID-19 vaccine schemes in the world. At the time of writing, roughly 89 per cent of Cubans of all ages were fully vaccinated, compared to just over 67 per cent in the US.[15] You could see this as a political statement, or you could see it as an invitation to consider that a different way of organising our lives is possible. But you should definitely view the lack of amplification of the Cuban vaccination programme as a deeper commentary on where the people who have most power in the global system believe the solutions to our most urgent problems will come from.

To date, it is unclear whether, if or even how the Cuban vaccination could create billionaires in a country where collective ownership of public resources is the law—it would be unfair to speculate on that given that history is replete with examples of how nominally socialist or communist countries have miraculously created billionaires. But what is objectively clear is that Cuba has modelled a path towards the development and distribution of crucial medicines that doesn't fundamentally function as a transfer of wealth from the poor and most vulnerable to people who are already wealthy. The trajectory of Cuba's vaccination programme compared to the various European programmes is really a challenge to the stories we are told about how certain injustices are a necessary part of the march towards progress, whatever that means.

But it's also a lesson to poor countries that are now trying to beef up their own vaccination programmes to be ready for the next pandemics. Making and distributing medicines should not be a pathway towards accumulation for its own sake. There is no private science of medicine. Making and distributing medicines in the modern era is always going to be a collaborative process that involves a lot of public money. That creates an obligation for those who are developing these medicines to make sure that they are available as widely as possible. The US and the West have failed at this dramatically. The decision to turn vaccines into a commercial product to be distributed at the maximum price to those who can pay the most has not just cost the US and Europe, it has cost the world. It set back the global vaccination project by months, allowing the disease to fester and mutate, and the emergency period to drag on indefinitely. We are increasingly desensitised to what death at this scale means, so let's write it out in full.

At the time of writing, at least 6.3 million people had died of COVID-19. That's 6,300,000 human lives. At least 5 million of those deaths occurred after the UK gave authorisation for the first COVID-19 vaccine to be distributed in the country, in December 2020. A different way is possible. It has to be. This cannot be the future of medicine.

17

SURVIVE

I am interested in how a human survives all this. I'm not sure we've grasped how much grief we are holding in our bodies and in our societies. By August 2022, at least 1 million people had died of the coronavirus in the United States, and almost 2 million across Europe, according to official governmental figures. I think the entire process of navigating the pandemic has hit many people harder than they may realise themselves. There are so many personal sadnesses, but there are also so many collective sadnesses that we haven't really had a chance to mourn properly. Grief accumulates in the personal and in the collective body. So many of us had no choice but to keep moving, even when it didn't make any sense. So many of us were forced to grieve privately and endure or simply move on. Where is all this grief supposed to go?

What about the grief over things that we haven't quite figured out how to mourn? How do we mourn all those people who deteriorated so quickly that there wasn't really time to process that death was on its way? I think about the Indians subjected to images of loved ones burning on funeral pyres in parking lots, because the crematoriums were too full. I think about countries like Ecuador, where people had to leave the bodies of the people they loved in the streets, because the morgues were overwhelmed. I think about all the people who had to say goodbye to friends and family from behind plastic curtains or over the phone, because the hospitals became too dangerous. I think about all the things doctors, nurses, the people who clean our hospitals and the people who make sure that all the procedures run on time have seen in the last three years—the impossible weight of grief and anger that they must be carrying, with no outlet. We were told that the only thing we needed to fear and mobilise around was death. But what are we supposed to do with these experiences and these things that we have seen?

I think many of us have had to come to terms with a sense of abandonment, and, significantly, with having been abandoned by the systems that are supposed to be in place to protect us. What is government for if it will not help those who are most vulnerable in times of great danger? After a deluge of promises about solidarity and sacrifice, it became very clear early in the pandemic that many of us were simply surplus to the demands of "the Economy", that amorphous entity to which all other wills must be bent. People with disabilities. People with chronic illnesses. People born African, or Asian. These people could not return to normal quite so quickly. How do we mourn when the tragedy has not only settled but also still feels impending?

I've written about grief at scale before because it became so common in my country, where we lost so many people to all kinds of mass violence. Anyone who has survived loss will tell you that you don't really get over it, you just grow accustomed to its weight. It becomes less of a sharp cut and more of a constant dull ache. The momentum for "normal" seems to be rushing us past the weight of what we have collectively experienced. But what was so great about normal, anyway, that means we must rush to return to it? Normal was never particularly kind for too many of us: shouldn't this be an opportunity to reset our relationship with these injustices? Shouldn't the goal be to rebuild better instead of just rebuilding "normal"? It is certain that there will need to be an "after". But I remain uncertain if that "after" should be "normal".

18

LONG COVID

The people who are suffering from it say that it feels like a permanent fog has settled over your mind and your body. As early as 2020, many who recovered from the pandemic said that they felt like the virus had never really left their bodies. Like there was a life before, and then there was a life afterwards, and there's a veil of some kind that allows you to see the before but not really access it. The brain fog can be bad enough to fundamentally change the way a person processes scents: food ends up smelling like rotting waste, things that were once pleasant end up smelling like garbage. It can also mean forgetting routine things, or losing the ability to focus on a task for extended period of time. Chronic fatigue can make it impossible to undertake the most banal tasks.[1] People who used to run marathons and who exercised daily have found it difficult to get out of bed in the morning.

The first symptom of COVID-19 for many people was a loss of smell and taste—the initial indicator that the virus was somehow interacting with our nervous systems. But there are also many things that science is still working to understand: why men are more likely to be hospitalised for the condition than women, or why women are more likely to suffer with Long COVID than men, for example.[2] COVID-19 has forced scientists to go back to the study of neurological conditions like fibromyalgia, which show similar patterns in the general population. But for observers, the failure to properly research gender differences in COVID-19 and fibromyalgia has been another reminder that science disproportionately focuses on the male experience of illness, rather than the female. More broadly, the people who emerged from the coronavirus with Long COVID had to fight to get onto the research and policy agenda. We were all so focused on not-dying we forgot to look into what was happening to those who survived. We were all so focused on preventing death that the experiences of those who lived were put on the back burner, perhaps to our collective detriment.

The speed with which the idea that COVID-19 was just a bad flu took root and spread across the world is an interesting case of how information travels and bends to the prevailing interests. People who suffered from the Long COVID said early on that they felt that they had been side-lined or ignored. Would it have been alarmist to make sure that people had all the information about Long COVID, in the same way as they were told about washing their hands or keeping their masks on?

19

PATENTLY UNJUST

THE CASE FOR GLOBAL VACCINE JUSTICE

In March 2021, the Kenyan government launched its vaccination plan for the country. At that time, the government, according to its own documents, aimed to vaccinate only 30 per cent of Kenya's population of roughly 48 million people—just citizens over fifty, those that work in health and in hospitality (tourism is a major earner for the country), and those with comorbidities. The government was clear: there is no proposal for the rest of us, no aspiration even to ensure that enough people are vaccinated to achieve "herd immunity".

All of this would have been egregious enough if it weren't happening against the backdrop of perhaps the worst display of national selfishness from wealthy countries in modern history. The European Union, the United States and Canada hoarded the vaccine, entering agreements to pre-purchase enough doses for up to six times their population in some cases. Moreover, because of national agreements with the pharmaceutical companies, they are also buying these doses at preferential prices (see Chapter 16). Poor countries are paying more for the scraps that remain after rich countries have had their fill.[1]

In fact, wealthy nations are using lifesaving interventions to play diplomacy. In 2021, the US, for example, ordered at least 300 million doses of the AstraZeneca jab—enough for at least one jab to almost its entire population—but the vaccine got stuck in Food and Drug Administration (FDA) approvals, and was still not approved for domestic use at the time of writing.[2] There were at least 7 million "releasable doses" available by March 2021, then White House press secretary Jen Psaki told the media, with another 30 million expected to be ready at the beginning of April that year.[3] Yet the US had ordered enough Moderna and Pfizer vaccines that it actually did not need the AstraZeneca doses. Instead of freeing up the existing doses, the government first promised to loan a paltry 4 million to Canada and Mexico. Following a large wave of criticism, it then pledged to share 60–80 million doses with the world, before backtracking on this due to the lack of FDA authorisation.[4] Billions of lives have been put at risk because rich countries have stood in the way of making vaccines more freely available, threatening to compound the already exacerbating inequalities. For contrast, by July 2022, 85 per cent of Canada's population of 38 million had received at least one jab, while only 3.45 million people in the Democratic Republic of the Congo (population 89.5 million) had had one or more vaccine shots. By May 2022, US pharmacies, states, territories and federal agencies had discarded at least 82.1 million doses of the vaccine—around a sixth of the total number distributed across the entire African continent up to that point.[5]

Meanwhile, the COVAX initiative led by the World Health Organization, designed to make global access to vaccines more equitable by coordinating countries to buy only enough vaccines for 20 per cent of their populations (so that at least all healthcare workers in the world could be vaccinated), struggled to procure enough jabs to meet demand. COVAX has purchased most of its doses from India (which produces 60 per cent of all jabs worldwide), but between April and September 2021, as the third wave of the virus battered the world's vaccine factory, this country put in place export controls to prioritise its domestic vaccination campaign. There's an injustice embedded in expecting Indian companies to continue to vaccinate the world in the middle of a national crisis, even as European and North American companies sitting on obscene surpluses explicitly refused to share.

Rich countries were slow to support COVAX, and Canada even actively undermined it by joining as a recipient, thereby making whatever scarce doses the initiative acquired even scarcer.[6] At the time the two most effective vaccines were made by Moderna and Pfizer, but Moderna refused to join COVAX until December 2021, while Pfizer only initially committed 40 million vaccine doses to the initiative.

Countries like China and Russia have also been making vaccines, which are less effective, but which scientists say are effective enough. The UK's then foreign minister Dominic Raab, however, declared in March 2021 that he would prefer African countries not get help from China or Russia, and instead to wait until Western countries were done with their vaccines.[7] No word on what the people whose lives were under threat were supposed to do while they wait, even as new waves of the virus and more lethal variants continued to take root across the continent.

I'm not sure how to describe what it feels like to be one of the millions—perhaps billions—of people for whom there was no plan. "Abandonment" only scratches the surface of being condemned to possible death by international greed and human folly. Here, at the intersection of cruel profiteering and woefully mediocre national and international government, is human life. We are not abstract figures or statistics. We are people, with families that we love and hopes for our futures that are being deliberately endangered by governments playing politics with lifesaving interventions.

But ours are not demands for pity. We are demanding justice. For one, the science affirms that without a global vaccination strategy, it doesn't matter how many doses rich Western countries hide away. This disease will not go away, and many people even in those countries will die. A 2020 study by the Global Vaccines Alliance (Gavi) found that if an 80 per cent–effective vaccine was distributed equitably based on the size of the population in each country, 61 per cent of global deaths could be prevented. This would compare to only 33 per cent of global deaths if rich countries were allowed to stockpile jabs. And this trend of averting more fatalities simply by making medicines equitably available would hold for less-effective vaccines like the Chinese Sinovac, too, with a jab with only 65 percent efficacy preventing 57 per cent of global deaths if allocated equitably, versus 30 per cent if hoarded.[8] The best way to save millions of lives around the world is to distribute vaccines fairly.

Early in the pandemic, poor countries that have the capacity to develop these vaccines have asked for manmade rules on intellectual property to be set aside in order to slow and halt the global emergency. At the end of 2020, India and South Africa petitioned the World Trade Organization (WTO) to waive intellectual property rights so that manufacturers in those countries could fill the gap in production capacity, but were denied.[9] Profits over people. At the WTO in 2021, the South African delegation had reminded participants that "developing countries have advanced scientific and technical capacities ... and that the shortage of production and supply [of vaccines] is caused by the rights holders themselves who enter into restrictive agreements that serve their own narrow monopolistic purposes putting profits before life." The head of the Africa CDC, Dr John Nkengasong, told the US House Foreign Affairs Committee in March 2021 that about six centres across Africa had the capacity to manufacture COVID-19 vaccines.[10]

Even though medicines are sequences of chemicals that are often made public, international rules on intellectual property prohibit manufacturing generic drugs unless the company or person who licensed it offers a waiver at the request of the country where they are registered. The WTO has an agreement called the Trade-Related Aspects of Intellectual Property Rights (TRIPS) that penalises manufacturing which violates the intellectual property rights of patent holders, and poor countries had asked governments that are party to this agreement to suspend its provisions to allow factories in their countries to produce the drugs without fear of penalty. After twenty months of negotiation, characterised by tough organised action from the Global South (and fantastic organisation from health rights activists) and unwillingness to concede by the wealthier countries, international governments eventually came to a limited agreement at the WTO in June 2022. It allowed several minor exceptions to intellectual property laws for a period of five years, but failed to issue a true intellectual property waiver. Médecins Sans Frontières described it as a "disappointing" pact that did not "address pharmaceutical monopolies or ensure affordable access to lifesaving medical tools, and will set a negative precedent for future global health crises and pandemics".[11]

In June 2021, the WHO Africa division helped coordinate an mRNA vaccine developing hub in Cape Town, and invited the main European and American companies—Moderna, Pfizer and AstraZeneca—to allow their researchers to collaborate with the facility to copy these vaccines. The companies did not respond to the WHO's invitation.[12] In February 2022, a South African company, Afrigen Biologics and Vaccines, finally managed to do exactly that: they reverse-engineered a version of Moderna's mRNA vaccine.[13] In March that year, Moderna eventually committed to not enforcing its patents, walking back on a policy to "reserve the right to do so in future once the disease became endemic" after significant public pressure.[14]

In December 2021, South African business Aspen Pharmacare also signed an agreement with vaccine manufacturer Johnson & Johnson to produce a coronavirus vaccine using drug substances supplied by the US pharmaceutical firm, becoming the first company licensed to distribute its own COVID-19 jabs in Africa. But by the time the plant was opened, African countries were so flooded with donations of leftover vaccines, often with close expiry dates that could not be effectively administered on time, that there was very little demand for Aspenovax. Aspen Pharmacare had not received a single order since licensing the jab, and the Africa CDC feared that the company may be forced to halt production.[15] Importantly, the Johnson & Johnson vaccine had suffered significant repetitional harm in the US. In May 2022, the US CDC had issued a warning restricting the administration of the drug for fear of dangerous blood clots, even though by their own admission, the benefits of the vaccine far outweighed these risks.[16] If you're not paying attention, you might think this is a story that proves that Africans didn't want to buy vaccines. But if you look closely, you'll see familiar patterns of hoarding and dumping that have killed other African industries like textiles or publishing.

This cycle of allowing commercial interests to outweigh human kindness has happened before. The same fights occurred during the last major novel pandemic, when rich countries refused to allow the production of life-saving anti-retroviral drugs to stop the mass deaths of HIV-positive people in poor countries.[17] While they argued about maintaining their profit margins, millions of people around the world died. In 1996, fully 10.5 per cent of Kenyans—literally one in every ten people— were living with HIV/AIDS.[18] I remember a time in Kenya when it felt like every family had lost a loved one to the disease, all while pharmaceutical giants fought to secure their bottom line. It is a reminder that something can be legal and still be unjust.

In the end, poor countries like Brazil, India and South Africa ignored the intellectual property claims of Western companies to produce generic drugs, but still came under tremendous political pressure, especially from the United States, which filed a complaint with the WTO that it eventually withdrew because of public criticism. This is why it is important to fight the injustice at the WTO.

Promises to donate doses of vaccines once all people in rich countries have been inoculated do not undo the injustice. There is a perverse logic embedded in the international order that cannot fathom equality, and needs poor countries on their knees in order to validate the feelings or perhaps even the existence of rich countries. It also shows us that there is a comprador class within poor countries allied with foreign capital. It would be disingenuous not to acknowledge the role that some African governments have played in the current situation, even while African regional coordination has been a stellar example for the world. The Kenyan government's vaccine plan, for example, is woefully insufficient, even while it continues to borrow heavily to fund legacy infrastructure projects that the country does not want or need, instead of focusing on managing and ending the pandemic.

In several African countries, the COVID-19 pandemic has been riddled with allegations of corruption and misappropriation of public funds. In September 2020, Kenya's Ethics and Anti-Corruption Commission released a report indicating that there had been "irregular expenditure" of 7.8 billion Kenyan shillings (US $65 million) of public funds in a procurement scandal at the state-run Kenya Medical Supplies Agency (KEMSA), which was to oversee the purchase of PPE in the country.[19] In South Africa, then health minister Zweli Mkhize was put on leave in June 2021 after allegations about the irregular allocation of communications contracts in support of the pandemic.[20] Other countries, including Malawi, Uganda, Cameroon and Nigeria have also been hit with accusations of corrupt dealing.

But these domestic failures in themselves do not explain the global inequality of outcomes when it comes to vaccines. First, even within Africa, these countries are outliers. Most African nations, to date, have no corruption scandals associated with their pandemic responses, and instead have faithfully, if sometimes slowly, allocated resources to tackling COVID-19. More importantly, pandemic corruption is not a uniquely African problem. In April 2021, international anti-corruption watchdog Transparency International found that one in five PPE contracts allocated by the UK government as part of their coronavirus response contained "one or more red flags for possible corruption".[21] And yet, at that point, around 57 per cent of people over twelve years old in the UK had already received at least one vaccine; this figure had risen to over 93 per cent by the time of writing. Indeed, according to *The Lancet*, by mid-2020, the UK had secured five bilateral deals for 270 million doses of vaccine, or enough for 225 per cent of its population.[22] Yet, the UK also paid £71 million for 27 million vaccine doses from COVAX, and in April 2021, it received 500,000 doses of the Pfizer-BioNTech vaccine through this initiative.[23] It's not enough to simply point to corruption as the reason why African countries do not have access to vaccines.

In fact, there was a global traffic jam in the vaccine supply chain, with manufacturers unable to keep up with the global demand. In large part this is because rich Western countries broke the agreement to begin by vaccinating frontline healthcare workers around the world before opening up vaccination to the general population. What will it mean now that rich countries have diverted some of that capacity towards the manufacture of booster shots, while more than a quarter of the world hadn't even received a single vaccine dose at the time of writing?

COVAX was supposed to be a fairness-pause, an opportunity to give all countries a fighting chance in the context of the anthems of global solidarity that were being sung during the worst of the outbreak in the West. In August 2021, China promised 2 billion doses of its vaccines to the world by the end of that year, of which 110 million were bought by COVAX, plus a US $100 billion donation to the initiative. By the end of that year, 1.3 billion doses had been distributed to low- and middle-income countries—the majority sold, not donated. While China has certainly helped to plug the supply chain gaps, more needs to be done. We needed a fairness pause, but in the medium term, the easiest way to ease up this traffic jam would be to make it possible for more countries to make vaccines. Cuba led the way by making its vaccine technology more freely available, but the Gamaleya Institute (the makers of the Russian Sputnik V vaccine) also promised in February 2021 to share their technology with manufacturers in Argentina. This is a big part of the multipronged strategy that African countries—and, indeed, other countries like India—are advocating. Waiving patent rights would allow countries with manufacturing capacity to copy the formulae for the vaccines without fear of punishment.

It is perfectly valid, and, indeed, crucial, to demand accountability from corrupt governments. Domestic activists in Africa are already doing that because we cannot let governments off the hook for the theft and the waste. But these demands will come to naught if rich countries keep on using charity as an excuse for injustice. We cannot demand that our governments reprioritise spending towards the purchase of vaccines if there are no vaccines to buy. And we cannot save the lives that are still under threat if we are only expected to wait for leftovers.

I could at this stage offer an elaborate explanation of how the West has jeopardised its soft power in the developing world by acting in such a brazenly selfish way. But I believe that we are living with the consequences of trying to make justice arguments through the lens of geopolitical ambition. If people structure their arguments by the rules of the game, then they validate those rules, even if they are inherently unjust. The idea that the only reason to help people in a crisis is to consolidate another country's power is part of the reason why conflicts in countries like the Central African Republic, which have little geo-strategic value to the imperialist powers, are getting lost. It is inhumane and ultimately counterproductive to collapse into this fallacy. Rich countries are hoarding vaccines because they hope to play politics with them. Meanwhile, people are dying.

Instead, my argument is a values-based one. Help people because they are people, not because it might help you. We must do the right thing, the just thing, because values must still matter. And while I have no idea how the pandemic will continue to play out in Africa, we will keep on living because we must. And we will keep on speaking out because all we can do is demand justice in this morally bankrupt system.

20

NECESSARY, RIGHTEOUS RAGE

I have to hold on to African American writer Audre Lorde's reflections on the uses of anger as I write this. Anger is a useful sentiment, and anger in the face of injustice is a human response. I've been known to make *kumbayah* statements in my life and work because, fundamentally, I want to believe that a world defined by justice and inclusion is possible, even in the face of staggering amounts of evidence that a critical mass of people simply does not want that reality to come to pass. So many of us are taught to make ourselves unfeeling of our anger as children because we are warned of its destructive nature. Anger can lead to rash judgments. Anger can lead to violence. Anger can lead to words uttered too quickly that can never be taken back. But Lorde reminds us that anger can be productive: "Focused with precision it can become a powerful source of energy serving progress and change".[1] Anger, sharpened by clarity and aimed at a deserving target, can lay waste to the things that obscure our perception of reality.

Let this anger lay waste to the myths that prevent us from reaching out for a different way of being.

Every African you know who has been paying attention to the world in the time of COVID-19 is angry, and justifiably so. Perhaps not since the HIV/AIDS pandemic first tore through our families and our communities have we been shown such callous disregard for our wellbeing from so many quarters and in so many different ways. Of course, we all knew on some level that the world was deeply unjust; that anti-black racism was an organising principle in so much of our international system; that when push came to shove, we were fundamentally on our own. But knowing this doesn't make it any easier to wade through the detritus of life since December 2019. Knowing that there was a risk on the horizon is nothing compared to living through the materialisation of that risk as systemic violence towards you, towards people who look like you, and towards people who hold the same passport as you.

To whom must this anger be directed so that it doesn't sit in our bones and make it impossible to see what needs to be done?

Perhaps the people who make and distribute medicine globally, who have learnt nothing in the nearly forty years since the start of the HIV/AIDS pandemic about the consequences of withholding drugs from people in order to make money? Providing healthcare is one of the basic principles and functions of entering a society. So, a system that allows citizens of poor countries to spend nearly three years, throughout the worst public health crisis in a generation, begging for medicine has failed? What appropriate reaction is there, outside of anger, for leaders who would rather let billions of perfectly good vaccines expire instead of allowing them to be distributed to the people who need it? What do we do with a system that sees the distribution of medicine as another opportunity to make a point about international power, instead of an opportunity to make a point about what it means to be human? What can one make of a politics that would turn medicine into a shortcut to accumulation?

NECESSARY, RIGHTEOUS RAGE

Anger is the only appropriate response. Not just for the inequality, but for the way demands for fairness were treated as abstract noise from people who should have known that they were going to get screwed over and should have responded accordingly. The demand was not for donations. The demand was for fairness, a cliché that has been spewed from all angles as the only true solution to so many inequalities in the world. We can have fairtrade bananas and fairtrade coffee, but this stops at fairly traded medicine? Will there ever be any historical account-ability for the decisions by wealthy countries to promise fairness through the COVAX scheme, only to turn around and short-change the global supply so dramatically in the heart of the emergency? What would that even look like? What are people supposed to do with all this anger while we wait to find out?

Perhaps the anger should be directed at the people who claim to be leaders on our continent? There are leaders like President Paul Biya of Cameroon, who squandered most of the money that was supposed to be used to protect his people against COVID-19. There are those who could not stop fighting each other long enough to allow a proper public health response. There are lead-ers in countries like Kenya or Uganda who spent more time sending the police to beat their citizens in the name of lock-downs than showing necessary leadership. And then there are those like the leaders of Tanzania and Madagascar, who put their populations squarely in harm's way by first denying the existence of the disease and then advocating for unproven and untested solutions. So, we level some of our anger at the people who claim to lead in our name but have only compounded the harm that we have been subjected to. Good leadership is supposed to be a buffer to defend us from the kind of unchecked greed and hoarding that we have witnessed since vaccines were first discov-ered. In too many places on the continent, that buffer failed.

Some of this anger has to be levelled in that direction.

149

But our anger must not overpower the many people without whose leadership and foresight the entire situation would have probably been worse. Without the leadership of Dr John Nkengasong and his colleagues at the Africa CDC, the lessons from the 2014 Ebola outbreak at a continental level might not have been consolidated and learnt from. Scientists and researchers from across the continent have made so many key contributions to the development of strategies and medicines to fight this new disease. There are several countries where governance worked the way it was supposed to, and our anger should not allow us to skip over that.

Even so, we should remain angry at the national leaders who believed so strongly in the myth that they could survive this crisis on their own that they broke apart the systems built to foster international cooperation. We are so angry at the countries which wrongly decided that because they did not need cooperation to survive, cooperation itself was unnecessary. It was not enough for them to hoard and jostle and steal. They also struck at the heart of the platforms which were supposed to bring people together to fix the problem. The global response to the COVID-19 pandemic, if we can even claim that there was anything global about it, failed, not because it had to, but because those with power decided that staking the future of the many on the potential survival of the few was a worthwhile risk.

We never wanted pity. We only wanted fairness. Our anger is because we have been the targets of sermons on global justice and fairness for decades, because our countries' politics and polices have been ripped apart in classrooms and boardrooms as examples of how not to do it. Many grand theories about what it means to live in the world together have been promoted over many years. But when it came to walking the walk, we were treated like disposable people. Where can we go to be treated fairly?

Racism is at the heart of these failures. There's no point in sugar-coating it or tiptoeing around it. The momentum around

COVID-19, as with the HIV/AIDS pandemic before it, was to act quickly only while it was a challenge to predominantly white countries. When the tragedy reached Africa, suddenly it became "inadvisable" to market the medicine that could keep people alive or to take coordinated action to suppress the contagion.

Lorde told us that "anger expressed and translated into action in the service of our vision and our future is a liberating and strengthening act of clarification, for it is in the painful process of this translation that we identify who are our allies with whom we have grave differences, and who are our genuine enemies."[2] If nothing else, this season of rage has demonstrated how all types of people and institutions perceive the value of some lives. We disagree with those allies who use pity to lobby for our survival because they see these demands differently to us. We wanted justice, not pity. And what Lorde calls genuine enemies, who come in various flavours, did not hesitate to invite death and suffering upon us.

If the future we want is one of freedom and justice, then it is important to sit with this clarifying anger and think soberly about what we want the world to look like if and when this emergency passes. Sitting with anger is not a pleasant experience; allowing rage to be expressed in order to call out those who claim to be our friends for having failed the tests of friendship is a disorienting and weighty process. But there is no way forward without it. There is no "normal" without it, and there is no "after" without it. Every African you know who has been paying attention to the global COVID-19 response is angry. Listen to us as we tell you why.

ACKNOWLEDGEMENTS

Some of these articles were previously published on various platforms. Sincerest thanks to all the editors who reviewed this work including Amy Hall, Mariya Petkova, Birce Bora, Kristina Rapacki, Christopher Shay, Oli Stratford and all their teams.

NOTES

FOREWORD

1. Albert Camus, *The Plague*, London: Penguin Classics, 2020 (new edition), trans. by Robin Buss, p. 208.
2. Ibid., p. 44.

1. REASONING BY ANALOGY: A STORY IN THREE ACTS

1. Shu Ting Liang, Lin Ting Liang and Joseph M Rosen, "COVID-19: a comparison to the 1918 influenza and how we can defeat it", *Postgraduate Medical Journal*, May 2021, vol. 97, no. 1147, pp. 273–4, http://dx.doi.org/10.1136/postgrad-medj-2020–139070 (last accessed 28 July 2022).
2. BBC News, "President Trump calls coronavirus 'kung flu'", 24 June 2020, https://www.bbc.com/news/av/world-us-canada-53173436 (last accessed 28 July 2022).
3. BBC News, "Li Wenliang: 'Wuhan whistleblower' remembered one year on", 6 February 2021, https://www.bbc.com/news/world-asia-55963896 (last accessed 28 July 2022).
4. Fred Andayi, Sandra S. Chaves and Marc-Alain Widdowson, "Impact of the 1918 influenza pandemic in coastal Kenya", *Tropical Medicine and Infectious Disease*, 2019, vol. 4, no. 2, https://doi.org/10.3390/tropicalmed4020091 (last accessed 28 July 2022).

5. Felix Tih, "Madagascar leader urges use of supposed COVID-19 cure", Anadolu Agency, 18 May 2020, https://www.aa.com.tr/en/africa/madagascar-leader-urges-use-of-supposed-covid-19-cure/1844564 (last accessed 28 July 2022).

6. Emmanuel Onyango, "Stephen Karanja: Kenyan anti-vaccine doctor dies from Covid-19", BBC News, 30 April 2021, https://www.bbc.com/news/world-africa-56922517 (last accessed 28 July 2022).

7. Janice Hopkins Tanne, "Covid 19: US government committee hears how social media spreads misinformation", *BMJ*, 2021, vol. 375, no. 2834, https://doi.org/10.1136/bmj.n2834 (last accessed 28 July 2022).

8. Frantz Fanon, "Concerning Violence", in *The Wretched of the Earth*, 1961. Available online at: http://www.openanthropology.org/fanonviolence.htm (last accessed 5 August 2022).

9. Jimoh Mufutau Oluwasegun, "Managing Epidemic: The British Approach to 1918–1919 Influenza in Lagos", *Journal of Asian and African Studies*, 2015, vol. 52, no. 4, pp. 412–24, https://doi.org/10.1177%2F0021909615587367 (last accessed 28 July 2022).

10. Ibid.

11. Josephine Ma, "Coronavirus: China's first confirmed Covid-19 case traced back to November 17", *South China Morning Post*, 13 March 2020, https://www.scmp.com/news/china/society/article/3074991/coronavirus-chinas-first-confirmed-covid-19-case-traced-back (last accessed 28 July 2022).

12. John Otis, "COVID-19 Numbers Are Bad In Ecuador. The President Says The Real Story Is Even Worse", NPR, 20 April 2020, https://www.npr.org/sections/goatsandsoda/2020/04/20/838746457/covid-19-numbers-are-bad-in-ecuador-the-president-says-the-real-story-is-even-wo?t=1659033878824 (last accessed 28 July 2022).

13. Ibid.

14. UN Development Reports, "Human Development Insights", no date, https://hdr.undp.org/data-center/country-insights?c_src=CENTRAL&c_src2=GSR&gclid=CjwKCAjw7cGUBhA9EiwArBAvoihMhKZ-v7uYo0DaClH4ntT3zR-I7UisqS1HgPmnuXFCH_te0tgGHBoCJmMQAvD_BwE&utm_source=EN&utm_medium=GSR&utm_content=US_UNDP_PaidSearch_Brand_English&utm_campaign=CENTRAL#/ranks (last accessed 28 July 2022).

15. Joe Myers and Rosamond Hutt, "This visualization shows you 24 hours of global air traffic—in just 4 seconds", World Economic Forum, 12 June 2016, https://www.weforum.org/agenda/2016/07/this-visualization-shows-you-24-hours-of-global-air-traffic-in-just-4-seconds/ (last accessed 28 July 2022).

16. Nathan Diller, "British airlines to drop mask mandates as U.K. lifts remaining travel restrictions", *The Washington Post*, 14 March 2022, https://www.washingtonpost.com/travel/2022/03/14/british-airlines-lift-mask-mandate/ (last accessed 28 July 2022).

17. Ibid.

2. LOCKDOWN

1. Eugenia Tognotti, "Lessons from the History of Quarantine, from Plague to Influenza A", *Emerging Infectious Diseases*, 2013, vol. 19, no. 2, pp. 254–9, https://doi.org/10.3201/eid1902.120312 (last accessed 28 July 2022).

2. Joshy Jesline, John Romate, Eslavath Rajkumar and Allen Joshua George, "The plight of migrants during COVID-19 and the impact of circular migration in India: a systematic review", *Humanities and Social Sciences Communications*, 2021, vol. 8, no. 231, https://doi.org/10.1057/s41599–021–00915–6 (last accessed 28 July 2022).

3. Carol Gitobu, "The shift to mobile technology for amplified government and humanitarian cash and voucher assistance amid the COVID-19 pandemic in Kenya", GSMA, 18 March 2021, https://www.gsma.com/mobilefordevelopment/blog/mobile-technology-government-humanitarian-cva-covid19-kenya/ (last accessed 8 August 2022).

4. National Institute for Communicable Diseases, "South African Scientists on the Inside Story of Discovering Omicron—and What Their Experience Offers the World about Future Variants. Podcast", 4 February 2022, https://www.nicd.ac.za/south-afri-can-scientists-on-the-inside-story-of-discovering-omicron-and-what-their-experience-offers-the-world-about-future-variants-podcast/ (last accessed 28 July 2022).

3. MASKING

1. World Health Organization, "Mask use in the context of COVID-19", 1 December 2020 (last updated), https://www.who.int/publications/i/item/advice-on-the-use-of-masks-the-community-during-home-care-and-in-health-care-settings-in-the-context-of-the-novel-coronavirus-(2019-ncov)-out-break (last accessed 28 July 2022).

2. Kar Keung Cheng, Tai Hing Lam and Chi Chiu Leung, "Wearing face masks in the community during the COVID-19 pandemic: altruism and solidarity", *The Lancet*, 16 April 2020, https://doi.org/10.1016/S0140–6736(20)30918–1 (last accessed 29 July 2022); Centers for Disease Control and Prevention, "Types of Masks and Respirators", 28 January 2022 (last updated), https://www.cdc.gov/coronavirus/2019-ncov/prevent-getting-sick/types-of-masks.html (last accessed 29 July 2022).

3. Dyani Lewis, "Why the WHO took two years to say COVID is airborne", *Nature*, 6 April 2022, https://www.nature.com/articles/d41586–022–00925–7 (last accessed 29 July 2022).

4. Centers for Disease Control and Prevention, "Types of Masks

and Respirators", 28 January 2022 (last updated), https://www.cdc.gov/coronavirus/2019-ncov/prevent-getting-sick/types-of-masks.html (last accessed 29 July 2022).

5. NTV Kenya, "Kibera: Tailor sews face masks for free distribution to the poor", (via YouTube), 3 April 2020, https://www.youtube.com/watch?v=1CLsfMffVrM (last accessed 29 July 2022).

6. Standard Digital Videos, "Activist Boniface Mwangi confronts police for allegedly harassing Korogocho dwellers", (via YouTube), 28 April 2020, https://www.youtube.com/watch?v=wS3iqGf6U4U (last accessed 29 July 2022).

4. UNMASKING

1. John Fritze and Michael Collins, "As Trump touts increased production, coronavirus swabs made during his Maine factory tour will be tossed in the trash", USA Today, 5 June 2020, https://eu.usatoday.com/story/news/politics/2020/06/05/trump-maine-puritan-throw-away-coronavirus-swabs/3153622001/ (last accessed 24 August 2022).

2. John-Allan Namu and Tess Riley, "Nine weeks of bloodshed: how brutal policing of Kenya's covid curfew left 15 dead", The Guardian, 23 October 2020, https://www.theguardian.com/global-development/2020/oct/23/brutal-policing-kenyas-covid-curfew-left-15-dead (last accessed 9 August 2022).

5. WAITING TO BE SAVED

1. Cultural Survival, "COVID-19 Awareness in Maa", (via Soundcloud), 26 April 2020, https://soundcloud.com/culturalsurvival/covid-19-awareness?utm_source=clipboard&utm_medium=text&utm_campaign=social_sharing (last accessed 29 July 2022).

2. Bruce Berman and John Lonsdale, Unhappy Valley: Conflict in Kenya & Africa, Ohio University Press, 1992, Chapter 2.

6. AIRBORNE

1. Fortune Business Insights, "Air Conditioners Market Size, Share & Industry Analysis, By Type ..., By Application ..., By Technology ..., By Distribution channel ... and Regional Forecast, 2022–2029", no date, https://www.fortunebusinessinsights.com/air-conditioners-market-102556 (last accessed 29 July 2022).
2. Maria Godoy, "Better air in classrooms matters beyond COVID. Here's why schools aren't there yet", NPR, 14 March 2022, https://www.npr.org/sections/health-shots/2022/03/14/1086125626/school-air-quality (last accessed 28 July 2022).
3. United States Environmental Protection Agency, "Indoor Air Quality: What are the trends in indoor air quality and their effects on human health?", 7 September 2021 (last updated), https://www.epa.gov/report-environment/indoor-air-quality#:~:text=Americans%2C%20on%20average%2C%20spend%20approximately,higher%20than%20typical%20outdoor%20concentrations (last accessed 29 July 2022).
4. Dimosthenis A. Sarigiannis (ed.), "Combined or multiple exposure to health stressors in indoor built environments", World Health Organization (Regional Office for Europe), October 2013, https://www.euro.who.int/__data/assets/pdf_file/0020/248600/Combined-or-multiple-exposure-to-health-stressors-in-indoor-built-environments.pdf (last accessed 29 July 2022).
5. Fanon, "Concerning Violence", op. cit.

7. GLOBAL

1. Aryeh Mellman and Norman Eisen, "Addressing the other COVID crisis: Corruption", Brookings, 22 July 2020, https://www.brookings.edu/research/addressing-the-other-covid-crisis-corruption/ (last accessed 29 July 2022).
2. Frantz Fanon, *The Wretched of the Earth*, 1961, chapter 3.

Available online at: https://www.marxists.org/subject/africa/fanon/pitfalls-national.htm (last accessed 9 August 2022).

3. BBC News, "Covid: Millions of vaccine doses destroyed in England", 25 February 2022, https://www.bbc.com/news/health-60506579 (last accessed 9 August 2022).

4. Mickey Djuric and Laura Osman, "Canada has thrown away at least one million COVID-19 vaccine doses: informal survey", CTV News, 19 November 2021, https://www.ctvnews.ca/health/coronavirus/canada-has-thrown-away-at-least-one-million-covid-19-vaccine-doses-informal-survey-1.5672817 (last accessed 29 July 2022).

5. House Foreign Affairs Committee, "Update on COVID-19 in Africa", (via YouTube), 17 March 2021, https://www.youtube.com/watch?v=xqw_89_xGb8 (last accessed 29 July 2022).

6. BBC News, "Coronavirus: EU stops short of vaccine export ban", 26 March 2021, https://www.bbc.com/news/world-europe-56529868 (last accessed 29 July 2022).

7. Justin Spike, "Hungary first in European Union for vaccinations, and deaths", AP News, 29 March 2021, https://apnews.com/article/pandemics-europe-viktor-orban-coronavirus-pandemic-china-0b4eea6c2757d2d16b8e5782c65ce418 (last accessed 29 July 2022).

8. Michael Camuñez, "America's coming vaccine glut: who should get it first", CNN, 16 March 2021, https://edition.cnn.com/2021/03/15/opinions/america-coming-vaccine-glut-mexico-camunez/index.html (last accessed 29 July 2022).

9. Mely Caballero-Anthony, "COVID-19 in Southeast Asia: Regional pandemic preparedness matters", Brookings, 14 January 2021, https://www.brookings.edu/blog/order-from-chaos/2021/01/14/covid-19-in-southeast-asia-regional-pandemic-preparedness-matters/ (last accessed 29 July 2022).

10. Jacque Wilson, "Borders closing over Ebola fears", CNN, 22 August 2014, https://edition.cnn.com/2014/08/22/health/ebola-outbreak/index.html (last accessed 29 July 2022).

11. Ibid.

12. Africa CDC, "AMSP opens COVID-19 vaccines pre-orders for 55 African Union Member States", 19 January 2021, https://africacdc.org/news-item/amsp-opens-covid-19-vaccines-pre-orders-for-55-african-union-member-states/ (last accessed 29 July 2022).

13. Seth Berkley, "COVAX explained", Gavi, 3 September 2020, https://www.gavi.org/vaccineswork/covax-explained (last accessed 29 July 2022).

14. David McAdams et al, "Incentivising wealthy nations to participate in the COVID-19 Vaccine Global Access Facility (COVAX): a game theory perspective", *BMJ Global Health*, 2020, vol. 5, issue 11, http://dx.doi.org/10.1136/bmjgh-2020–003627 (last accessed 29 July 2022).

15. Kate Elder, "COVAX: A broken promise for vaccine equity", Médecins Sans Frontières, 21 February 2022, https://www.doctorswithoutborders.org/latest/covax-broken-promise-vaccine-equity (last accessed 29 July 2022).

16. Emily Ashton, "U.K. Set to Scrap Covid Hotel Quarantines as Soon as Tuesday", Bloomberg UK, 13 December 2021, https://www.bloomberg.com/news/articles/2021-12-13/u-k-set-to-scrap-red-list-hotel-quarantines-as-soon-as-tuesday (last accessed 29 July 2022).

17. Shoshana Kedem, "#UNGA: African leaders call for additional IMF SDRs for pandemic recovery", *African Business*, 23 September 2021, https://african.business/2021/09/economy/unga-african-leaders-call-for-additional-imf-sdrs-for-pandemic-recovery/ (last accessed 29 July 2022).

18. International Monetary Fund, "Special Drawing Rights (SDRs)", no date, https://www.imf.org/en/Topics/special-drawing-right (last accessed 29 July 2022).

19. International Monetary Fund, "2021 General SDR Allocation", 23 August 2021 (last updated), https://www.imf.org/en/Topics/special-drawing-right/2021-SDR-Allocation (last accessed 29 July 2022).

8. POLICING A PANDEMIC

1. Amnesty International, "Amnesty International Report 2020/21: The State of the World's Human Rights", 2021, https://www.amnesty.org/en/wp-content/uploads/2021/06/English.pdf (last accessed 11 August 2022).
2. BBC News, "Kenya policeman charged with murder after curfew killing of teenager", 23 June 2020, https://www.bbc.com/news/world-africa-53150397 (last accessed 11 August 2022).
3. ADF, "Kenyan Police Under Scrutiny After Lockdown Deaths", 7 September 2021, https://adf-magazine.com/2021/09/kenyan-police-under-scrutiny-after-lockdown-deaths/ (last accessed 28 July 2022).
4. Victor Oluoch, "Deadly force: Unlawful killings by police still prevalent in Kenya", Nation, 5 October 2019 (last updated 13 April 2021), https://www.nation.co.ke/newsplex/2718262–5299758–12jlxhhz/index.html (last accessed 29 July 2022).
5. Fanon, "Concerning Violence", op. cit.
6. Namu and Riley, "Nine weeks of bloodshed ...", op. cit.

10. THE ART OF ASKING USEFUL QUESTIONS

1. United Nations, "68% of the world population projected to live in urban areas by 2050, says UN", 16 May 2018, https://www.un.org/development/desa/en/news/population/2018-revision-of-world-urbanization-prospects.html (last accessed 11 August 2022).

11. DEATH AND FUNERAL ANNOUNCEMENTS

1. Robyn Kriel and Briana Duggan, "Kenya covers up military massacre", CNN, 31 May 2016, https://edition.cnn.com/2016/05/31/africa/kenya-soldiers-el-adde-massacre/index.html (last accessed 29 July 2022).

2. BBC News, "Somalia's al-Shabab killed '180 Kenyan troops' in el-Ade", 25 February 2016, https://www.bbc.com/news/world-africa-35658500 (last accessed 29 July 2022).

3. Stephanie Nolen, "Trying to Solve a Covid Mystery: Africa's Low Death Rates", *The New York Times*, 23 March 2022, https://www.nytimes.com/2022/03/23/health/covid-africa-deaths.html (last accessed 29 July 2022).

4. Freda Kreier, "Morgue data hint at COVID's true toll in Africa", *Nature*, 23 March 2022, https://www.nature.com/articles/d41586–022–00842–9 (last accessed 29 July 2022).

5. National Aids Control Council, "Kenya HIV Estimates, Report 2018", October 2018, https://nacc.or.ke/wp-content/uploads/2018/11/HIV-estimates-report-Kenya-20182.pdf (last accessed 11 August 2022).

12. DISPOSABLE PEOPLE

1. Centers for Disease Control and Prevention, "About Dengue: What You Need to Know", 23 September 2021 (last reviewed), https://www.cdc.gov/dengue/about/index.html#:~:text=Each%20year%2C%20up%20to%20400,40%2C000%20die%20from%20severe%20dengue (last accessed 11 August 2022).

2. World Health Organization, "Malaria", 26 July 2022, https://www.who.int/news-room/fact-sheets/detail/malaria (last accessed 29 July 2022).

3. Dan Cohen, "Op-Ed: Why a PPE shortage still plagues America and what we need to do about it", CNBC, 22 August 2022, https://www.cnbc.com/2020/08/22/coronavirus-why-a-ppe-shortage-still-plagues-the-us.html (last accessed 29 July 2022).

4. GlobalData Healthcare, "Lack of protective equipment preparation led to spike in frontline healthcare worker deaths", Medical Device Network, 21 May 2020, https://www.medi

caldevice-network.com/comment/healthcare-worker-deaths-covid-19/ (last accessed 29 July 2022).

5. Canada Institute for Health Information, *Pandemic Experience in the Long-Term Care Sector: How Does Canada Compare With Other Countries?*, Ottawa, ON: CIHI; 2020. Available online at: https://www.cihi.ca/sites/default/files/document/covid-19-rapid-response-long-term-care-snapshot-en.pdf (last accessed 11 August 2022).

6. The COVID Tracking Project, "Long-Term-Care COVID Tracker", 7 March 2021 (last updated), https://covidtracking.com/nursing-homes-long-term-care-facilities (last accessed 11 August 2022).

7. Ibid.

8. International Long-Term Care Policy Network, "International data on deaths attributed to COVID-19 among people living in care homes", 22 February 2022, https://ltccovid.org/2022/02/22/international-data-on-deaths-attributed-to-covid-19-among-people-living-in-care-homes/ (last accessed 29 July 2022).

9. Charlotta Stern and Daniel B. Klein, "Stockholm City's Elderly Care and Covid19: Interview with Barbro Karlsson", *Society*, vol. 57, no. 4, pp. 434–45, https://doi.org/10.1007/s12115-020-00508-0 (last accessed 11 August 2022).

10. Ibid.

11. Johan Ahlander and Niklas Pollard, "Sweden failed to protect elderly in COVID pandemic, commission finds", Reuters, 15 December 2020, https://www.reuters.com/article/health-coronavirus-sweden-commission-idUSKBN28P1PP (last accessed 29 July 2022).

12. Kerry Dobransky and Eszter Hargittai, "People with Disabilities During COVID-19", *Contexts*, November 2020, vol. 19, issue 4, pp. 46–9, https://doi.org/10.1177/1536504220977935 (last accessed 29 July 2022).

13. Office for National Statistics, "Updated estimates of corona-

virus (COVID-19) related deaths by disability status, England: 24 January to 20 November 2020", 11 February 2021, https://www.ons.gov.uk/peoplepopulationandcommunity/births-deathsandmarriages/deaths/articles/coronaviruscovid19relateddeathsbydisabilitystatusenglandandwales/24januaryto20november2020 (last accessed 29 July 2022).

14. Tom Shakespeare, Florence Ndagire and Queen E. Seketi, "Triple jeopardy: disabled people and the COVID-19 pandemic", The Lancet, 16 March 2021, vol. 397, issue 10282, pp. 1131–3, https://doi.org/10.1016/S0140–6736(21)00625–5 (last accessed 29 July 2022).

15. May Bulman and Helen Hoddinott, "'It's a lovely awakening': Elderly people and children sing and dance together in UK's first intergenerational care home", The Independent, 25 March 2018, https://www.independent.co.uk/news/uk/home-news/elderly-children-intergenerational-care-home-nightingale-house-a8271876.html (last accessed 29 July 2022).

13. VOCABULARIES

1. Abigail Beall, "The heart-wrenching choice of who lives and dies", BBC News, 29 April 2020, https://www.bbc.com/future/article/20200428-coronavirus-how-doctors-choose-who-lives-and-dies (last accessed 29 July 2022).

2. Edwine W. Barasa, Paul O. Ouma, Emelda A. Okiro, "Assessing the hospital surge capacity of the Kenyan health system in the face of the COVID-19 pandemic", PLOS One, 20 July 2020, vol. 15, no. 7, https://doi.org/10.1371/journal.pone.0236308 (last accessed 19 August 2022).

15. OMICRON

1. Zoe Flood, "Inside the Botswana lab that discovered Omicron", Al Jazeera, 14 December 2021, https://www.aljazeera.com/

features/2021/12/14/inside-the-botswana-lab-that-discovered-omicron (last accessed 19 August 2022).

2. Tim Lister and David McKenzie, "How South African scientists discovered Omicron and set off a global chain reaction", CNN, 2 December 2021, https://edition.cnn.com/2021/12/02/world/south-africa-omicron-origins-covid-cmd-intl/index.html (last accessed 11 August 2022).

3. Marnie Hunter and Forrest Brown, "Latest US travel rules: What you need to know about the changes prompted by Omicron", CNN, 30 December 2021, https://edition.cnn.com/travel/article/new-us-travel-rules-omicron-what-to-know/index.html#:~:text=Yes%2C%20as%20of%2012%3A01,Namibia%2C%20South%20Africa%20and%20Zimbabwe (last accessed 29 July 2022).

4. Raf Casert, "New 'omicron' variant prompts global travel restrictions", PBS, 26 November 2021, https://www.pbs.org/newshour/world/new-virus-variant-detected-in-south-africa-prompting-global-travel-restrictions (last accessed 11 August 2022).

5. DW, "COVID: Germany confirms first 2 cases of omicron variant", 27 November 2021, https://p.dw.com/p/43ZrT (last accessed 11 August 2022).

6. Reuters, "Omicron variant was detected in the Netherlands before S. Africa flights", 30 November 2021, https://www.reuters.com/business/healthcare-pharmaceuticals/omicron-variant-was-detected-netherlands-before-s-africa-flights-2021-11-30/#:~:text=AMSTERDAM%2C%20Nov%2030%20(Reuters),Amsterdam's%20Schiphol%20airport%20on%20Nov (last accessed 11 August 2022).

7. Camus, *The Plague*, op. cit., p. 43.

16. THE NUMBERS ON THAT

1. Oxfam, "Ten richest men double their fortunes in pandemic while incomes of 99 percent of humanity fall", 17 January 2022,

https://www.oxfam.org/en/press-releases/ten-richest-men-double-their-fortunes-pandemic-while-incomes-99-percent-humanity (last accessed 29 July 2022).

2. Juliana Kaplan, "Billionaires have added $1.3 trillion to their net worths during the pandemic—a 44% increase from March 2020", Business Insider, 25 February 2021, https://www.businessinsider.com/billionaires-added-13-trillion-net-worths-during-pandemic-wealth-inequality-2021–2?r=US&IR=T (last accessed 11 August 2022).

3. Sarah Johnson, "Covid created 20 new 'pandemic billionaires' in Asia, says Oxfam", The Guardian, 14 January 2022, https://www.theguardian.com/global-development/2022/jan/14/covid-created-20-new-pandemic-billionaires-in-asia-says-oxfam (last accessed 11 August 2022).

4. Anne Trafton, "Explained: Why RNA vaccines for Covid-19 raced to the front of the pack", MIT News, 11 December 2020, https://news.mit.edu/2020/rna-vaccines-explained-covid-19–1211 (last accessed 29 July 2022).

5. Dan Diamond, "The crash landing of 'Operation Warp Speed'", Politico, 17 January 2020, https://www.politico.com/news/2021/01/17/crash-landing-of-operation-warp-speed-459892 (last accessed 29 July 2022).

6. Samuel Cross et al, "Who funded the research behind the Oxford–AstraZeneca COVID-19 vaccine?", BMJ Global Health, 2021, no. 6, http://dx.doi.org/10.1136/bmjgh-2021–007321 (last accessed 29 July 2022).

7. Jon Cohen, "South Africa suspends use of AstraZeneca's COVID-19 vaccine after it fails to clearly stop virus variant", Science, 8 February 2021, https://www.science.org/content/article/south-africa-suspends-use-astrazenecas-covid-19-vaccine-after-it-fails-clearly-stop (last accessed 15 August 2022); KEMRI and Wellcome Trust, "ChAdOx1 nCOV-19 Vaccine Trial—Frequently Asked Questions about the Trial", no date, https://kemri-wellcome.org/news/chadox1-ncov-19-

vaccine-trial-frequently-asked questions-about-the-trial/ (last accessed 29 July 2022).

8. Owen Dyer, "Covid-19: Countries are learning what others paid for vaccines", *BMJ*, 2021, vol. 372, no. 281, https://doi.org/10.1136/bmj.n281 (last accessed 29 July 2022).

9. Ryan Cross, "Moderna reaped more than $12 billion in profits from COVID vaccine sales last year", *The Boston Globe*, 24 February 2022 (last updated), https://www.bostonglobe.com/2022/02/24/business/moderna-reaped-more-than-12-billion-profits-covid-vaccine-sales-last-year/ (last accessed 11 August 2022).

10. Pharmaceutical Technology, "Moderna reports $18.5bn total revenue in full-year 2021", 25 February 2022, https://www.pharmaceutical-technology.com/news/moderna-reports-revenue-2021/ (last accessed 11 August 2022).

11. Official website of Elizabeth Warren, "Warren, Merkley, and Jayapal Lead Colleagues in Urging the Biden Administration to Review Moderna-HHS Contract and Expand Global COVID-19 Vaccine Access", 13 October 2021, https://www.warren.senate.gov/newsroom/press-releases/warren-merkley-and-jayapal-lead-colleagues-in-urging-the-biden-administration-to-review-moderna-hhs-contract-and-expand-global-covid-19-vaccine-access (last accessed 11 August 2022).

12. Katerini T. Storeng and Antoine de Bengy Puyvallée, "Why does Pfizer deny the public investment in its Covid-19 vaccine?", International Health Policies, 3 December 2020, https://www.internationalhealthpolicies.org/featured-article/why-does-pfizer-deny-the-public-investment-in-its-covid-19-vaccine/ (last accessed 11 August 2022).

13. The Russian Government, "Government lowers maximum sales price for Sputnik V vaccine", 25 February 2021, http://government.ru/en/news/41609/ (last accessed 15 August 2022); Sputnik Vaccine, "The Russian Direct Investment Fund (RDIF)", no date, https://sputnikvaccine.com/about-

us/the-russian-direct-investment-fund/ (last accessed 29 July 2022).

14. Sara Reardon, "Cuba's bet on home-grown COVID vaccines is paying off", *Nature*, 22 November 2021, https://www.nature.com/articles/d41586–021–03470-x (last accessed 29 July 2022).

15. Our World in Data, "Coronavirus (COVID-19) Vaccinations", (updated daily), https://ourworldindata.org/covid-vaccinations?country-OWID_WRL (last accessed 11 2022.

18. LONG COVID

1. Centers for Disease Control and Prevention, "Long COVID or Post-COVID Conditions", 11 July 2022 (last updated), https://www.cdc.gov/coronavirus/2019-ncov/long-term-effects/index.html (last accessed 29 July 2022).

2. David Cox, "Why are women more prone to long Covid?", The Guardian, 13 June 2021, https://www.theguardian.com/society/2021/jun/13/why-are-women-more-prone-to-long-covid (last accessed 29 July 2022).

19. PATENTLY UNJUST: THE CASE FOR GLOBAL VACCINE JUSTICE

1. Owen Dyer, "Covid-19: Countries are learning what others paid for vaccines", *BMJ*, 2021, vol. 372, no. 281, https://doi.org/10.1136/bmj.n281 (last accessed 29 July 2022).

2. Aakash B, Guy Faulconbridge and Kate Holton, "U.S. secures 300 million doses of potential AstraZeneca COVID-19 vaccine", Reuters, 21 May 2020, https://www.reuters.com/article/us-health-coronavirus-astrazeneca%20%20%20idUSK-BN22X0J9 (last accessed 29 July 2022).

3. CBC News, "White House says U.S. plans to send 1.5 million doses of AstraZeneca vaccine to Canada", 18 March 2022,

https://www.cbc.ca/news/politics/reuters-us-canada-mexico-vaccine-1.5954871 (last accessed 29 July 2022).

4. Carmen Paun, "Biden drops AstraZeneca vaccine from latest donation", Politico, 21 June 2021, https://www.politico.com/news/2021/06/21/biden-astrazeneca-vaccine-donation-scrapped-495342 (last accessed 15 August 2022).

5. Joshua Eaton, "The U.S. has wasted over 82 million Covid vaccine doses", NBC News, 6 June 2022, https://www.nbcnews.com/news/us-news/covid-vaccine-doses-wasted-rcna31399 (last accessed 3 August 2022).

6. Darren Major and Catherine Cullen, "Canada shouldn't take vaccine doses from COVAX partnership, says Canada's former UN envoy", CBC News, 26 February 2021, https://www.cbc.ca/news/politics/canada-stephen-lewis-covax-1.5930344 (last accessed 29 July 2022).

7. Jill Lawless, "UK: Poorer nations should get 'gold-standard' COVAX vaccines", AP News, 1 March 2021, https://apnews.com/article/coronavirus-pandemic-ivory-coast-824ac282d-9b26bea6d1664797470551e (last accessed 15 August 2022).

8. Priya Joi, "Equitable COVID-19 vaccine distribution will lead to the biggest reduction in deaths", Gavi, 4 November 2020, https://www.gavi.org/vaccineswork/equitable-covid-19-vaccine-distribution-will-lead-biggest-reduction-deaths (last accessed 15 August 2022).

9. Ann Danaiya Usher, "South Africa and India push for COVID-19 patents ban", *The Lancet*, 5 December 2020, vol. 396, issue 10265, pp. 1790–1, https://doi.org/10.1016/S0140–6736(20)32581–2 (last accessed 29 July 2022).

10. House Foreign Affairs Committee, "Update on COVID-19 in Africa", (via YouTube), 17 March 2021, https://www.youtube.com/watch?v=xqw_89_xGb8 (last accessed 29 July 2022).

11. Médecins Sans Frontières, "Lack of a real IP waiver on COVID-19 tools is a disappointing failure for people", 17 June 2022, https://www.msf.org/lack-real-ip-waiver-covid-19-

tools-disappointing-failure-people (last accessed 15 August 2022).

12. Amy Maxmen, "South African scientists copy Moderna's COVID vaccine", *Nature*, 3 February 2022, https://www.nature.com/articles/d41586-022-00293-2 (last accessed 29 July 2022).

13. Ibid.

14. Jamie Smyth, Hannah Kuchler and Andres Schipani, "Moderna vows never to enforce Covid jab patents in policy U-turn", *Financial Times*, 7 March 2022, https://www.ft.com/content/425ec5ad-1ae0-4460-a588-6aadfe5d52d6 (last accessed 29 July 2022).

15. Paul Adepoju, "Lack of orders could halt COVID-19 vaccine production in South Africa", Devex, 14 April 2022, https://www.devex.com/news/lack-of-orders-could-halt-covid-19-vaccine-production-in-south-africa-103052 (last accessed 29 July 2022).

16. US Food & Drug Administration, "Coronavirus (COVID-19) Update: FDA Limits Use of Janssen COVID-19 Vaccine to Certain Individuals", 5 May 2022, https://www.fda.gov/news-events/press-announcements/coronavirus-covid-19-update-fda-limits-use-janssen-covid-19-vaccine-certain-individuals (last accessed 29 July 2022).

17. Jacqui Wise, "Access to AIDS medicines stumbles on trade rules", *Bulletin of the World Health Organization*, 2006, vol. 84, no. 5, pp. 342–4, https://www.ncbi.nlm.nih.gov/pmc/articles/PMC2627352/ (last accessed 29 July 2022).

18. The Global Fund, "Kenya and Global Fund Sign New Grants to Accelerate Response to Diseases", 15 December 2017, https://www.theglobalfund.org/en/news/2017/2017-12-15-kenya-and-global-fund-sign-new-grants-to-accelerate-response-to-diseases/ (last accessed 15 August 2022).

19. Humphrey Malalo, "Kenya anti-graft agency slams procurement of COVID-19 equipment", Reuters, 24 September 2020,

https://www.reuters.com/article/us-kenya-corruption-idUSKCN26F3CC (last accessed 15 August 2022).

20. South African Government, "President Cyril Ramaphosa places Minister Zweli Mkhize on special leave", 8 June 2021, https://www.gov.za/speeches/president-cyril-ramaphosa-places-minister-zweli-mkhize-special-leave-8-jun-2021–0000 (last accessed 15 August 2022).

21. Transparency International UK, "Concern over Corruption Red Flags in 20% of UK's PPE Procurement", 21 April 2021, https://www.transparency.org.uk/track-and-trace-uk-PPE-procurement-corruption-risk-VIP-lane (last accessed 15 August 2022).

22. Ann Danaiya Usher, "A beautiful idea: how COVAX has fallen short", *The Lancet*, June 2021, vol. 367, no. 10292, pp. 232–2325, https://doi.org/10.1016/S0140-6736(21)01367-2 (last accessed 15 August 2022).

23. Ibid.

20. NECESSARY, RIGHTEOUS RAGE

1. Black Past, "(1981) Audre Lorde, 'The Uses of Anger: Women Responding to Racism'", 12 August 2012, https://www.blackpast.org/african-american-history/speeches-african-american-history/1981-audre-lorde-uses-anger-women-responding-racism/ (last accessed 29 July 2022).

2. Black Past, "The Uses of Anger ...", op. cit.